stay shArp

52 Ways to Keep Your Mind, Not Lose It

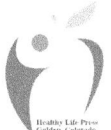

Healthy Life Press
Golden, Colorado

Dr. David B. Biebel
James E. Dill, MD
| AND |
Bobbie Dill, RN

stay shArp

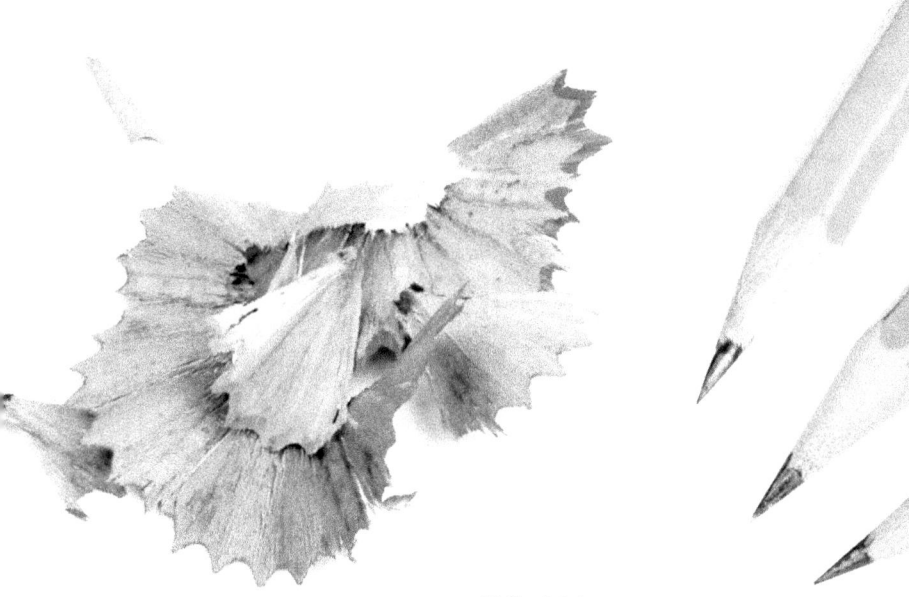

52 Ways to Keep Your Mind, Not Lose It

STAY SHARP: 52 Ways to Keep Your Mind, Not Lose It
Copyright © 2015 by David B. Biebel and Bobbie Dill

Authors   David B. Biebel, DMin
James E. Dill, MD
Bobbie Dill, RN

Designer   Judy Johnson

Published by:
Healthy Life Press • 9375 Blue Mountain Drive • Golden, CO 80403
www.healthylifepress.com

Printed in the United States of America

No part of this publication may be reproduced, stored in a retrieval system, or transmitted in any form or by any means—for example, electronic, photocopy, recording—without the prior written permission of the author, except for brief quotations in printed reviews.

Library of Congress Cataloging-in-Publication Data
Biebel, David B., Bobbie Dill
Stay Sharp: 52 Ways to Keep Your Mind, Not Lose It

ISBN 978-1-939267-60-3
1. Christian Living / Healthy Living; 2. Body, Mind & Spirit / Inspiration & Personal Growth

Most Healthy Life Press resources are available wherever books are sold. Distribution is primarily through www.SpringArbor.com, www.Amazon.com, www.deepershopping.com, and www.healthylifepress.com. Multiple copy discounts available directly from Healthy Life Press. Wholesale distribution is through www.SpringArbor.com (a division of www.IngramContent.com), and www.deepershopping.com. Our ePublications are available through www.Amazon.com (Kindle), www.BN.com (Nook), and for all eBook readers through www.deepershopping.com. Wholesale copies of our eBooks are also available through www.IngramContent.com (www.SpringArbor.com). Combination offers of printed and electronic books of the same title are available at a discount from the publisher at: www. healthylifepress.com. Most resources ordered directly from the publisher receive free shipping.

Unless otherwise noted, all Scripture quotations are taken from the *Holy Bible, New International Version*. Copyright © 1984, International Bible Society. Scripture marked KJV is from the *King James Version* of the Bible. Scripture marked NASB is taken from the *New American Standard Version*, Copyright© 1977, the Lockman Foundation. Scripture marked MSG is taken from *The Message*. Copyright © 1993, 1994, 1995, 1996, 2000, 2001, 2002. Used by permission of NavPress Publishing Group. Scripture marked NLT is taken from the Holy Bible, New Living Translation Copyright © 1996, 2004, 2007, 2013 by Tyndale House Foundation. Scripture marked CEV is from the Contemporary English Version. Copyright © 1995 by American Bible Society. All Scripture quotations used by permission.
All rights reserved.

For information on our products, or how to publish with us, e-mail: info@healthylifepress.com. Capitalization of pronouns related to deity follows The Christian Writer's Manual of Style (Grand Rapids: Zondervan, 2004).

This book is not intended to replace a one-on-one relationship with a qualified healthcare professional, but as a sharing of knowledge and information from the research and experience of the authors. You are advised and encouraged to consult with your healthcare professional in all matters relating to health. The publisher and authors disclaim any liability arising directly or indirectly from the use of this book. Authors' note: All stories in this book are true and used by permission. Most are disguised to protect the privacy of those involved. Stories may include composite characters.

This book is revised , expanded, and updated from *Your Mind at Its Best*, by the same authors.

Contents

Seven Pillars of Brain Health — 7
Dedication and Acknowledgements — 8
Introduction — 9

"Love Works Miracles" by Dr. Walt Larimore — 10

1. Stop Aiming and Shoot Already! — 13
2. To Sleep Perchance to Dream — 17
3. Why'd I Come in Here? — 21
4. Wow Your Brain — 25
5. Is this a Senior Moment, or . . . ? — 29
6. Bring Back the Slide Rule — 33
7. Just Dance — 37
8. Get Engaged — 41
9. Stop Killing Yourself Slowly — 45
10. Play Furniture Roulette — 49
11. A Concert State of Mind — 52
12. Stoke Your Belly Fire — 57
13. How Do You Want Your Change? — 61
14. A Funny Thing Happened on the Way to the Foramen — 65
15. Getting Your Marbles Back — 69
16. Brain Safe Your Home — 73
17. Eureka! — 77
18. Feed Your Gold Mind — 81
19. Don't Eat Squirrel Brains — 85
20. This is Your Brain on. . . . Any Questions? — 89
21. Stick to Quiet Fish — 93
22. Let's Go Surfing Now, Everybody's Learning How — 97
23. Participate by Proxy — 101
24. Fertilize Your Mind — 105
25. Eat the Rainbow — 109
26. Rot Not Thy Brain — 113
27. You Can Go Home Again — 117

28.	Stop and Smell the Memories	121
29.	Can You Say "Talafa Lava?"	125
30.	"Water, Water Everywhere . . . nor any drop to drink"	129
31.	Cardiphonia	133
32.	Bug Off	137
33.	You are Hard Wired for Joy	141
34.	Where the Past and Future Meet	145
35.	Buoy Your Amygdala	149
36.	The Secret of Your Senses	153
37.	Synaptic Serenades	157
38.	De-myth-ti-fying Brain Health	161
39.	Which Planet are You From?	167
40.	Unfoggin' Your Noggin'	171
41.	Toxic Shocks	177
42.	Unbind Your Mind	181
43.	This is Your Brain on Canvas	185
44.	Mind Your Head	189
45.	Go Beltless	193
46.	Listen to Your Other Brain	197
47.	Reinvent Yourself	201
48.	Play with Half a Glass	205
49.	Scrabble Your Brain	209
50.	Welcome to Club Med	213
51.	The Secret of Staying Focused	217
52.	In Spirit and in Truth	221

Conclusion: If Your Brain Could Talk	225

"Love Works Miracles" – The Rest of the Story	229
About the Authors	232
Notes	249
Healthy Life Press Resources	

Seven Pillars of Brain Health

Nutrition
Eat whole food that is as close to its natural state as possible; avoid food-like substances that come already prepared for your convenience.

Physical Exercise
Get off the couch, and take your brain for a walk . . . as often as possible.

Cognitive Exercise
Challenge your mind, for brain pain equals brain gain.

Rest
Reboot your mind daily; ordinarily, this is called "sleep."

Stress Management
Learn to experience peace of mind even in stressful situations, and thus relax your body, mind, and spirit.

Spirituality
"Instead of worrying, pray. Before you know it, a sense of God's wholeness, everything coming together for good, will come and settle you down" (Philippians 4:6-7, MSG).

Connection
To boost your brain power, nurture mutually supportive relationships.

Understand and practice these primary contributors to brain health and you'll be far more likely to keep your mind, not lose it.

Dedication

TO THE MEMORY OF DR. DAVID B. LARSON, A pioneer in the study of the relationship of faith to health, and to Dr. Harold G. Koenig, our friend, who carries forward the same banner.

Acknowledgments

WE WISH TO THANK SUE FOSTER (MA, LMFT) for her invaluable contribution to our efforts to produce this book.

We also wish to thank Gary Burlingame and Bruce Incze, whose textual contributions and research-based suggestions were so very helpful in relation to a number of chapters.

In addition, we wish to thank Betsy Dill for her help in assembling the "woodpile" for the chapter "Rejoice." We could not have produced this book as well without the help of all of you. Thank you!

Introduction

THESE DAYS PEOPLE ARE LIVING LONGER. BUT with longer life comes new fears, among them the fear of long, slow mental decline. No one wants to lose their mind; everyone wants to stay sharp.

Perhaps you picked up this book because you are looking for trustworthy information about achieving and maintaining optimal brain health. Perhaps you have experienced some "senior moments," and you want to slow, stop, or even reverse that trend. You may want to learn about ways to protect yourself and your family from habits of thinking or acting that might be diminish the best short-term and long-term functioning of your brains.

This book presents what can seem to be mystifyingly complex information in an easy-to-read, enjoyable, inviting, and sometimes even entertaining style. It's a chapter-by-chapter journey into the intricacies of the human brain—how it functions best, how to keep it healthy, how its health relates to your health in general, and the role of relationships and spirituality and other subjects not often discussed in a book on this subject.

Chapters are short, with practical tips offered following each. They are designed to stand alone, so you can focus on one per week if you wish, ignore some occasional informational overlap, and start anywhere you wish, because topics are arranged in no particular order.

Our biggest challenge in creating this book was not deciding what to include, but what to leave out, because in preparing to write we reviewed scores of books on relevant topics, and thousands of documents, including many research studies and Internet posts. The net result is a medically reliable, faith-based, lay-level digest of the best information available about how to sharpen your mind and keep it that way.

If you are seeking help and hope in the face of a diagnosis of brain injury or brain disease in yourself or someone you love, this book is for you. And to bolster your hope from the get go, we begin with a real-life true story that one of our good friends, Dr. Walt Larimore, has been kind enough to share. Most likely, whatever you're facing today is no greater obstacle than was overcome through this family's faith and love, coupled with God's healing grace. This story will help you see that, as challenging as your situation may be, it is much too early to give up.

"Love Works Miracles"
by Walt Larimore, MD

FOR THE FIRST SEVERAL YEARS OF OUR MARRIAGE, my wife Barb and I journeyed through medical school in New Orleans, a Queen's Fellowship in Great Britain, travels throughout Europe, and then we returned to the US for my residency at Duke University.

During my internship, in the autumn 1978, I was finishing a thirty-six-hour shift in the Emergency Room when Barb, who was thirty-six weeks pregnant, called. I could hear uncertainty in her voice. "I think my water bag broke."

Twenty-four hours later, Katherine Lee Larimore, all five pounds, fifteen and one-half ounces of her, was in our arms. She was four weeks premature, but to me she looked fabulous, incredible, marvelous and magnificent, amazing and astonishing, dainty and delicate, beautiful and brilliant. Quite objectively, I thought she was the most beautiful baby I had ever seen!

When Kate was two months old, Barb knew that something was wrong, as Kate was not progressing normally. Kate's doctor reminded us that Kate had been premature and that we might expect some delays—so I didn't worry.

To Barb, I seemed not only not to worry, but to her I seemed too busy to ever notice or care about her or Kate. As the pressures and time demands of my internship built, Barb felt alone and abandoned. By the time Kate was four months old, Barb was feeling even more frustrated, fearful, scared, and abandoned. Kate seemed to her to be falling further behind in her development.

Barb wondered: "What's going on? Why my child, God? Why can't I get any answers? I don't deserve this, Lord! What did I do to deserve this?" And, her prayers seemed only to bounce off a silent God.

When Kate was six months old, I confided with a friend who was a pediatrician: "Mary, I'd like to ask your opinion on a case. I have a friend with a baby who . . ."

She asked a few questions. She looked concerned.

"What do you think it is?" I inquired. She said—and her words echo in my ears as if she spoke them just yesterday—"Walt, it sounds to me like a case of cerebral palsy."

I was shocked. I felt the blood drain from my face and my eyes widen as I began to consider the implications of this diagnosis. The very wise pediatrician, tears in her eyes, took my hand in hers. "Walt," she almost whispered, "this baby is not just the baby of a friend is it?"

As tears streamed down my cheeks, through quivering lips, I cried, "No, it's our Kate."

A CT scan confirmed our fears. Kate's left brain was only half its normal size. Worse, on the right side there was no brain—nothing but water and a thin wispy scar where the right brain had been.

It hit me like a ton of bricks. All total, Kate had only 25 percent of a normal brain. The pediatric neurologist summed it up: "Walt and Barb, Kate will never walk. She'll never talk. She'll never be able to do any type of higher reasoning. You'll have to take care of her for life. Just take her home and love her the way she is."

We both cried and cried for weeks. The sunshine in our lives disappeared. The pit deepened. The path darkened. With the doctor's pronouncement, our hopes for Kate and for her life . . . our dreams and our desires were shattered.

And, worst of all, God was silent. He was completely silent. I couldn't hear him. I couldn't see him at work. Worst of all, I didn't trust that he was big enough or even cared enough to care for this problem.

Because I couldn't hear him, because I couldn't see him at work, because I was not able to fully trust him, my fear turned to anger. "God, how can you do this to me?"

"Why me, Lord?"

My escape became immersion in my work. I was angry at God. I was angry at Barb.

Before we knew it, we both were at the end of our strength. Our resources were exhausted. Our hopes and dreams had died, and our relationship was dying, also. But, just when we were at the end of our rope . . . when we seemed to have no other options . . . when there seemed to be no one to turn to but God himself . . . his work in our lives became unmistakable. He showed me he still loved me; he still wanted to guide and comfort me. He wanted me to know that he was trustworthy even when I am not.

One day while in my first year of family medical practice, I received an urgent message. My nurse said, "Walt, Barb just called and said you need to hurry home. No one is hurt, she just needs you at home, now."

Later in the book we'll come back to, as Paul Harvey used to say, "The Rest of the Story." But for now, we just wanted to plant this seed of hope in your mind, trusting it will grow and bear fruit as you read on.

And one other thing . . . when we have all agreed on something and speak as one, we'll say "we." When we are speaking for ourselves or from our own personal experience, versus analysis or comparison of data, we identify who is speaking.

Dave, Jim, and Bobbie

1

Stop Aiming and Shoot Already!

> *Every significant vital sign—body temperature, heart rate, oxygen consumption, hormone level, brain activity, and so on—alters the moment you decide to do anything . . . decisions are signals telling your body, mind, and environment to move in a certain direction."*   *– Deepak Chopra*

DECISIONS . . . DECISIONS. . . . IT SEEMS LIKE from the moment you wake to the moment you get back to sleep again maybe sixteen hours later, you're making decisions. Sometimes (usually toward the end of the workday when your energy is low) you may think that if anyone asks you to make one more decision, even about a relatively small issue (Shall I overnight this document or will Priority Mail be fast enough?) you will go barking mad.

Life is a series of decisions. Estimates differ on the number of decisions you make each day, but an educated guess would be about five thousand. This is approximately five decisions per minute over sixteen waking hours. That's 35,000 per week;

1,820,000 per year, and so forth. Most of these are fairly mundane, including what you choose to eat (over 200 decisions per day) or what you choose to wear (not as many decisions daily, unless you obsess over how you look). Should I take the umbrella? Should I fill up on fuel on the way to work or the way home?

Many decisions are made quickly: Shall I pass the car in front of me now, or wait? Should I respond to that text message that just came in from my child's school now, while I'm driving? And once in a while, there are bigger decisions that require a lot more time, concentration, knowledge, and wisdom: Should I take that job offer, even if it means moving the family 1,000 miles? Is it time to arrange assisted living for Mom, and if so, what kind of facility would be best for her? Shall we discontinue life-support for Grandma, even if some family members are not so sure we should do so?

The question is not if you will have to make decisions today, but how will you do so? While ordinary choices usually lead to ordinary consequences, even some decisions that seem quite ordinary (I will answer that text right now, despite the fact that I am driving) can have immediately disastrous results. Other mundane decisions, including what you have to eat day-by-day, can also have disastrous results, but those are more long-term, as in the development of chronic diseases related to obesity.

The following factors can affect your decisions and therefore the direction of your life:

- Lack of Rest: Is your brain rested enough to make this decision today? If you were up all night last night, studies suggest that you may be inclined to take more risks than usual. You've heard the phrase "sleep on it," in relation to decision making. Research suggests that your unconscious mind will keep working on the problem even as you sleep.[1]

- Low Blood Sugar: Your blood sugar vacillates throughout the day. Your brain needs glucose in order to function well. A study on "decision fatigue" found that a simple glucose fix (sugared lemonade, but not lemonade that was artificially sweetened): ". . . improved people's self-control as well as the quality of their decisions: they resisted irrational bias when making choices, and when asked to make financial decisions, they were more likely to choose the better long-term strategy instead of going for a quick payoff."[2]
- Your Psychological State: One article warned, "Depressed people . . . clearly have difficulty with value-based decision making: because nothing feels good or seems appealing, all options appear equally bleak and making choices becomes impossible."[3] When you are grieving is also not a good time to make decisions you might regret later, such as selling the house or the car for far less than they are worth just to get them off your mind, or moving away as soon as possible, which can affect your support system.[4]
- Impairment Due to Substances: Do not make important decisions when your thinking is impaired by any substance, including prescription medications. Mixing these with alcohol or other drugs leads to many extremely bad decisions, some of these capable of inflicting significant pain on those you really do love when you're sober.
- Prior Brain Injury: If you have experienced brain damage due to injury or illness, accept the likelihood that your decision-making abilities have been affected. For example, research shows that prior brain damage can make shopping (where you may have to make multiple decisions fairly quickly) difficult, due to the distraction

of so many options.[5] Risky decision making and impulsivity can also be a problem. It's best to have at least one trusted friend or counselor to provide feedback on your intended choices.

- Chronic Stress: One study showed that when you are experiencing chronic stress, you're likely to choose directions that are familiar even when a better choice is known to be available. This tendency is reversible as your stress is resolved or you learn to manage it well.[6]

Some programs promise to help you improve your decision-making abilities. For example, Dr. Daniel Amen (a leading brain health authority and author of multiple best-selling books on the subject) believes that his "One-Page Miracle for the Soul" can help you develop focus and improve your decision-making,[7] though the overall focus of his programs is on brain health in general and the benefits that come from that.

The bottom line on this subject is that good brain health is foundational to good decision making. In fact, good health in general, including your physical, emotional, relational, and spiritual health, is foundational to good decision making. You can build a trustworthy foundation by practicing the advice in this book's seven arenas of focus. You can also improve your decision-making abilities through specific brain-training programs.

SHARPER BRAIN TIPS

- Limit your information gathering to what you need in order to decide. Some people "shoot from the hip," making many decisions quickly and instinctively. Others aim, aim, aim, but are reluctant to pull the trigger until they believe they have all the data needed. Some get "stuck" in endless data gathering, which is one way to avoid making a decision. But not to decide is to decide, by default. When you have enough pertinent and trustworthy information, decide and move on.

- Learn to discern between crucial decisions and those that are not so crucial. Make the latter decisions more quickly, and save more of your decisionmaking energy for the former.

- If you're having trouble resolving a particularly difficult issue, solicit advice from a trustworthy source who has been in your situation and is willing to share insights gained.[8]

2

"To Sleep, Perchance to Dream"[1]

> *It is a common experience that a problem difficult at night is resolved in the morning after the committee of sleep has worked on it.*
> — John Steinbeck

Some people think of sleep as passive, and a few hard-driving folks may even resent the fact that in order to remain sharp they must exit the rat race on a daily basis and catch some Z's. Interestingly, though, the very thing they resent often provides a solution to a problem that has such folks stymied.

I (Dave) know by experience what John Steinbeck means about the "committee of sleep." Sometimes in writing or editing something, I'll hit a word wall inhibiting further progress. On many occasions over more than thirty years of wordsmithing, a nap or a good night's sleep has provided a solution that might not have occurred otherwise. It seems that while my body sleeps, my mind organizes what I've been thinking. And sometimes a solution has even come while dreaming.

By contrast, the loss of even one or two night's sleep can affect our cognitive abilities, as described by this neurosurgeon:

> "I was sleep deprived. So what? Still confident that there was nothing wrong with my ability to function at full capacity, I flew to San Francisco, where NASA's Ames Research Center keeps a full-size virtual-motion simulator of a Boeing 747 jumbo jet. After a few hours of training and several takeoffs and landings, I had mastered the 747—or so I thought.
>
> "My assignment was to stay awake to the point of sleep deprivation and then try to fly again. After 30 hours, I felt more exhausted than I could ever remember. Then I was back in the cockpit. Remarkably, all those simple landing sequences were suddenly much harder to remember. Just keeping the nose of the plane level was a real challenge. . . .
>
> "My experience, I learned, is hardly unique. A chronically sleep-deprived person will often go through repeated episodes of microsleep, sometimes accompanied by microdreams (which are usually interpreted as hallucinations). If you have been up for more than 20 hours, your reflexes are roughly comparable to those of someone [who is] legally drunk. . . ."[2]

An estimated 30 percent of American workers do not get enough sleep to function at peak performance, with the cost to companies they work for (in lost productivity) estimated at $63.2 billion annually.[3] Add to this the incalculable cost of workplace accidents, poor decision-making, auto accidents on the way to and from work, and the emotional dysfunction of workers (and managers) who are constantly exhausted, and you have a serious problem that is only recently getting the attention it deserves.

In general, people who are sleep-deprived have problems with drowsiness, concentration, memory, and cognitive functioning.[4] There is some evidence that sleep deprivation negatively affects the immune system as well. So here's a little quiz to help you assess your sleep needs. Check any statement that applies to you:

- _ I can only wake up early enough for my day with the help of an alarm clock.
- _ After waking, I find it hard to get up and get going.
- _ I often use the "snooze" button to get just a little more sleep.
- _ Often during the work week, I feel tired, irritable, or stressed.
- _ Concentrating for more than a few minutes is difficult.
- _ Sometimes I can't remember important things.
- _ I often feel like I'm in slow motion.
- _ I often fall asleep watching TV.
- _ I often fall asleep after a heavy meal.
- _ I often fall asleep after drinking just a small amount of alcohol.
- _ I often feel drowsy while driving.
- _ On weekends, I often sleep in until late in the morning.
- _ I seem to run out of energy most afternoons.

Results: If you check four or more of these questions, you probably need more sleep.[5]

Sleep may be the Creator's way of giving your brain time to repair itself from the work it did during the day. Without this time of rest and renewal, you neurons might not function as well as they should. At the same time, while you're sleeping your brain uses neurons that are not as active when you're awake, thus keeping them "exercised." Deep sleep may help the brain "file" memories, something like what you do when you quit working and file things you want to be able to find later.

In one study, one group memorized information before going to sleep. They were allowed to sleep deeply. When awakened their recall of the memorized information was significantly better compared with another group that memorized the same information, then had their deep sleep (dreaming time) interrupted by researchers.[6]

Dreams have intrigued humanity as far back as there has been sleep, the most intriguing question about them being, "What did that mean?" Dreams and their meaning play a significant role in the Bible, the Old Testament's Joseph being the most famous interpreter. Many times in biblical texts, the claim is made that one person or another received a message from God in a dream.

While the scientific jury is still out in relation to the meaning of dreams, or even what the specific function of dreaming is in relation to health in general, there is no doubt that the two hours that most adults spend dreaming each night are crucial to healthy brain function.

How much sleep do you need? Well, the largest study of its kind on longevity found that the "ideal" average number of hours of sleep for adults seems to be seven, though many sleep six and some eight, so a range of normal sleep is generally thought to be an average of six to eight hours per night. Much more or less than that and your system does not like it. Not only so, a five-year study of over 5,000 men and women aged forty-five to sixty-nine at baseline found that a change in one's average duration of sleep per night to less or more results in cognitive decline equivalent to three to eight years of aging.[7] So, while scientists try to figure out why this might be true, your best approach is to get an average of six to eight hours per night of sleep and to try to maintain that throughout your adult life.

SHARPER BRAIN TIPS

- Try to sleep an average of six to eight hours/night.
- For the next week, when you first wake up, ask yourself if you feel refreshed and renewed or tired—if tired, talk with your physician about it.
- Educate yourself about changes in setting or lifestyle that lead to restful sleep, and implement as many improvements as you can.[8]
- Place a high enough value on sleep that you feel zero guilt when you need it.
- If worry keeps you awake, and your thoughts go round and round, try listing the things that trouble you or that you're afraid you might forget, and leave that list on the bed stand until morning.

3

Why'd I Come in Here?

Memory moderates prosperity, decreases adversity, controls youth, and delights old age.   —*Anonymous*

See if this scenario describes something familiar: You're rushing to get ready to leave for work when you remember that before you leave, you want to set the timer on the washer and refill the cat's bowl of food. Still brushing your hair, you start walking toward the utility room. Just then, your cell phone rings, and you pause, half-way to your goal, in the middle of the living room, to take the call. When you disconnect, you look around the living room, searching for a clue to the question: *Why did I come in here?*

Memory is important to us not only because it catalogues our life events but also because being able to remember enhances our ability to think on higher levels. Although memory loss is not necessarily a *result* of aging, it can *accompany* that process. So it is prudent to discover and practice ways to keep our memory sharp as we age.

I (Bobbie) am laughing as I write this chapter because we just moved to yet another new apartment and we are struggling to memorize which drawer holds the silverware, which way to turn to find the bathroom in the middle of the night, and the location of all the light switches. Sounds easy, right? Trust us, it isn't! At least not when you have to do it multiple times every year.

Our phenomenal brains are not only capable of memorizing details of new surroundings, but of reconstructing past experiences. Whether you are attempting to learn to ride a bike, remember the beloved face of your great-grandmother, or find the silverware drawer, all of these challenges have two things that are necessary for success: learning and reconstructing the past. When we learn, a group of neurons fire at the same time, producing an experience. The neuronal pathway is changed so that in the future these same neurons are more likely to fire together. Repeating this cycle makes it easier to "recall" and reproduce the skill being learned.

Memories are made as we flow through the following steps. The first few seconds of storing a new memory take place in the sensory part of our brains, which automatically record touch, scent, taste, sound, or visual cues of the moment. Then the new memory is placed into short-term storage. Memories are stored in bits and pieces distributed throughout the brain. Each memory is made up of a web of sensory information and facts. Our memory "software" is created in such a way that it makes long-term memories less destructible. For instance, the memory of a beloved dog may be sparked when we see an animal of the same breed, and our mind is flooded with details about that doggie-friend that we thought were forgotten and gone.

Researchers have found that the hippocampus in the brain triggers this memory web of neurons that are emotionally charged or well-learned and retrieves the short- or long-term memory.[1]

The next phase is similar to triage in a medical setting. The hippocampus determines if a memory should be saved. Is it important to remember how many trees were swaying in the wind outside your window? Probably not. But what about how much computer paper is left? Yes, this should be retained at least long enough to make it to your shopping list. If a memory pathway is not strengthened it will quickly fade; it must be reinforced in order to eventually find its way into long-term storage where it will have staying power. If the memory is associated with a strong emotion like fear, or better yet, joy, it will be easier to retain. This is in part due to the body chemicals that are secreted during emotional times. High levels of stress or sleep deprivation, on the other hand, greatly impede our ability to remember.

The third phase of memory function is the retrieval phase. When we recall the memory, it comes back by way of the nerve pathways, and the more frequently we recall it, the better it is remembered. Most of us remember learning our multiplication tables, which have years of staying power, and most would agree the process was tinged with at least a low dose of stress!

Researchers have found that when we memorize new things it promotes neuron growth and actually creates new brain connections. The myelin sheaths that cover and protect our neural pathways are strengthened and the brain itself grows in size, giving us extra thinking capacity.[2]

The hippocampus is not only important in memory recall but also is crucial in navigation. When we move around, neurons (known as place cells) activate to tell us where we are. This process is known as spatial memory.[3] And its practice will help keep your mind sharp.

SHARPER BRAIN TIPS

- Clear away distractions and really focus on new information.
- Clear your mind by listening to music for a while with your eyes closed and no list nearby.
- Designate a place to keep your essential "gear."
- Review new information each day until the new information is entrenched in your memory bank.
- Choose one thing on your "to do" list and do it until it is done, then cross it off, celebrate, repeat.

4

Wow Your Brain

He who can no longer pause to wonder and stand rapt in awe, is as good as dead; his eyes are closed. – Albert Einstein

Until very recently, awe and wonder have been the realms of theology, philosophy, psychology, and the arts. With the advent of non-invasive brain imaging, however, these topics are now the subject of study by neuroscientists, who have been showing an increasing interest in the effect of awe on the brain.

Now that so many disciplines have their fingers in the "awe" and "wonder" pie, it is even more crucial to define terms. One group studying the question offers the following definitions: "Awe: a direct and initial feeling when faced with something incomprehensible or sublime. Wonder: a more reflective feeling one has when unable to put things back into a familiar conceptual framework."[1] So awe is the feeling (or sensation), and wonder is the response.

Scientists are discovering that the sensation of awe and the response of wonder are a key to a more fulfilling life. For example, Dacher Keltner, PhD, devotes much of his research to studying awe. "Cultivating awe," he says, "is part of unlocking the truest sense of life's purpose. With awe, it's not, 'Wow, that's a really tall dinosaur,'" he says. "It's, 'Wow, there's something bigger than me.'"[2]

From my own experience (Dave) all of my most awe-some times have happened in the wild. Many occurred while hiking in the Rockies, where awe and wonder are the only appropriate responses when you see what God made. Through the years, I've spent literally months in elk camp, at 10,000 feet in elevation, where the night sky is so clear that you feel you could almost touch the stars. When you lie back and gaze at that vista, you know deep inside that there is no way that all of this happened by chance. And even more wonder-full is the thought that the One who made it all actually cares personally for you.

The psalmist and former shepherd, David, expressed this same sense of awe and wonder: "When I consider Your heavens, the work of Your fingers, the moon and the stars, which You have ordained; what is man that You take thought of him, and the son of man that You care for him? Yet You have made him a little lower than God, and You crown him with glory and majesty!" (Psalm 8:3-5, NASB).

Scientific investigation of awe is in its infancy—an interesting description, for the scientists involved will do well if they can retain the perspective of infants, who express more wonder at their world than most people at any other age). Three studies rendered the following results, here quoted from an article's abstract: "When do people feel as if they are rich in time? Not often, research and daily experience suggest. However, three experiments showed that participants who felt awe, relative to other emotions, felt they had more time available and were less impatient. Participants who experienced awe also were more willing to volunteer their time to help other people, more strongly preferred experiences over material products, and experienced greater life satisfaction. Mediation analyses revealed that these changes in decision making and well-being were due to awe's ability to alter the subjective experience of time. Experiences of awe bring people into the present moment, and being in the present moment underlies awe's capacity to adjust time perception, influence decisions, and make life feel more satisfying than it would otherwise."[3]

While the identification of specific brain regions involved in experiencing awe awaits further study, it is clear that awe and wonder are gifts from the Maker, perhaps intended to connect us to the Larger Story, of which our lives are a part. This connection provides perspective on our day to day experience, including all the problems that can be the source of brain-killing stress—one antidote being the belief that God really does "have the whole world in his hands," including us.

The astronauts would have the best perspective on this, having actually experienced a "God's eye view" of the Earth. One of them, Jerry Ross, wrote:

> "I am an astronaut. In my life I have seen views of Earth and the universe from a perspective once known only to God. . . . I have launched into space seven times and ventured into the blackness of the universe on nine spacewalks. Seeing the beauty of Earth from orbit along with the enormity, the complexity, and the order of the universe strengthened my faith in a loving God who gave us a beautiful, fragile place to live.
>
> "I carried my Bible with me on my last flight. . . . I read the creation story in Genesis while preparing to go to sleep in the ISS [International Space Station]: 'When God began creating the heavens and the earth, the earth was at first a shapeless, chaotic mass, with the Spirit of God brooding over the dark vapors. Then God said, "Let there be light," And light appeared.'

"... reading the creation story in Genesis while looking down on the beauty of the Earth from space was a very powerful moment for me. Personally, I find it impossible to believe that everything I saw from space was created without God. Science explains many things. We understand more about the universe every day. But there are things that science will never be able to explain. To me, that is evidence of God's infinite wisdom and knowledge, and those things beyond our understanding are the things we can hope to have revealed in the life after death."[4]

In terms of awe and wonder, some things we know: Awe and wonder are good for the soul, so they are also good for your health in general. Things we have yet to discover: Whether these sensations are related to specific parts of the brain, or if, perhaps like spirituality, they involve and affect our most important organ more globally.[5]

SHARPER BRAIN TIPS

- Describe what you "see" in your mind's eye when you re-live a childhood time that was so wondrous, mysterious, and surprising that all your senses were fully alert and you felt totally alive. Include not only what you saw, but what you heard, smelled, felt, and tasted, if taste was involved.
- Then recall a similar experience you have had within the past ten years. How was it similar to that childhood event? How was it different?
- Review some of the things that have diminished your sense of awe and wonder. Write down the ways you have been affected, and what you might do to reverse that result.
- Find someone who will relive with you some of your most wonder-filled experiences. This could be a spouse, friend, colleague, or even a child. Ask that person to share their own stories with you.
- Ask yourself if you believe that regaining a sense of wonder would be good for your psychological, physical, sociological, or spiritual health.
- Gaze at a single flower for 15 minutes. Look under, over, and around the petals. If it's a tall flower, lie on you back with your head as far under the petals as possible, and see how this augments the experience.

5

Is This a Senior Moment ... Or?

Our brain creates our life: perception, movement, thought and emotion, memories, speech and intelligence are features of this extraordinary and most complex organ.
– Author Unknown

WE TREASURE OUR BRAIN AND ALL ITS ABILITIES, WHICH is why, when we begin to detect some slips and slides in memory we panic and maybe even wonder if we could have Alzheimer's. To avoid unnecessary worry and to guard our brain health it is important to know the facts and when, or if, we need to get a brain check-up.

Memory lapses are often caused by a lack of stimulation or not being fully engaged in life, which can result in a lag in forming new brain cells and pathways. Forgetting something we just learned yesterday is frustrating, but it's even worse when we can't remember something we've known for years! What we're trying to recall seems to be "on the tip of our tongue," but the brain's search for the right file in the neuronal archives turns up empty. And the harder we try to make ourselves remember, the more stubborn our "search engine" becomes. This plight not only disturbs us, but it can affect our friends as we turn to them with a plea for help only to find that they, too, have developed "amnesia" in relation to what our brain is searching for. When this occurs, our stress level may increase—for example if we're late for an important appointment, and we need to call the other person, but we simply can't remember that telephone number. And it seems that the harder we try, the worse it gets.

The phenomenon behind these occurrences takes place in the frontal lobe of our brain, which is very sensitive to stress hormones. When the frontal lobe (the keeper of stored memories) senses fight or flight situations, it shuts down to allow lower brain functions to use the energy. In other words, if your brain detects a dangerous or stressful situation it automatically ramps up the areas needed to keep you safe, in which case remembering your aunt's address is no longer a priority.

Of course that needed piece of information often pops back into your mind when it is no longer needed and you are working in the garden or drifting off to sleep! Dave had this experience recently, when he and his sister were visiting during a family reunion, and she was trying to recall the name of the fire chief in their town when they were kids. Neither could remember, hard as they tried. But when Dave was drifting off to sleep that very night, Mr. B's name came to his mind like magic.

As humorous as some "memory moments" can be, situations turn serious when memory lapses worsen or are combined with other symptoms. Dementia, including Alzheimer's, results in a gradual loss of cognitive function. Symptoms include memory loss, problems with focus, language, and problem-solving skills, difficulty controlling emotions and moods, and personality changes. Alzheimer's disease, the thief of memory, usually targets the hippocampus first and then spreads to other areas of the brain, slowly killing brain cells and incapacitating its victim.

In the past it was believed that genes were the key contributor to Alzheimer's, but now there are many more theories about what causes this disease. Among them are such things as immune dysfunction, metabolic conditions including obesity, insulin resistance and diabetes, overwhelming stress such as PTSD, environmental toxins, and nutritional deficiencies.

Scientists have shown that only about 4 percent of the population between ages sixty to seventy-four have Alzheimer's. But the figure jumps to almost 50 percent after age 85.[1] However, this progression is not inevitable.

For example, one study found that seniors who exercise and eat a Mediterranean-style diet seem to be at lower risk for Alzheimer's. This was recently confirmed by researchers at Columbia University when 1,880 septuagenarian New Yorkers were studied and those who followed the healthiest diets were 40 percent less likely to develop Alzheimer's. In addition those who got the most exercise were 37 percent less likely to develop the disease. The greatest benefit occurred for those who both ate healthfully and remained active. Those who scored high in both areas were 59 percent less likely to develop Alzheimer's.[2]

One physician-friend wrote, "I see dozens of folks per week who are mostly over 65 years of age. One of the most common fears expressed to me is that they are losing brain function in memory, in executive function, in their ability to control their own affairs in life. Not recalling a name that goes with a face or where they put their glasses or what they went into a room to get, are typical problems that set off these alarms. These symptoms do not suggest that dementia is just around the corner, but it takes a good bit of convincing to reduce that fear. It turns out that physical exercise does more to prevent brain shrinkage in the hippocampus area or to reduce strokes than mental exercises, so first I recommend that they keep their brains oxygenated by exercising regularly, while they also keep on playing bridge or chess or reading."

SHARPER BRAIN TIPS

In his book, *The Memory Cure*, Majid Fotuhi, MD, PhD, suggests these mental exercises to enhance your memory. The first letter of each exercise spells the word: ATTENTION.

- <u>Attention:</u> Focus all your senses on one issue.

- <u>Take notes:</u> Write down details about your tasks, places to go, people to see.

- <u>Try hard:</u> Use memorization techniques, categories, repetition, and store some things (keys, wallet, glasses, briefcase, etc.) in the same place day by day.

- <u>Emotions:</u> You are more likely to recall names and faces connected to events that affected you emotionally.

- <u>No fatigue, and no stress:</u> Long-term stress and fatigue can damage the hippocampus, hindering your memory.

- <u>Tease your brain:</u> Trying or learning new things exercises and strengthens your brain.

- <u>Imagination:</u> Vividly picture the items on a list you wish to memorize. The funnier or more ridiculous each image, the more likely you'll remember it.

- <u>Organization:</u> Every week, prioritize the coming week's agenda. Use index cards, computers, wall boards, or whatever works to keep your daily "to-do" list organized.

- <u>Never too late:</u> Old "dogs" can learn new tricks. Exercising your memory is a lot like exercising your muscles, and has a similar result—improved function. [3]

6

Bring Back the "Slide Rule"

Math is like going to the gym for your brain. It sharpens the mind. — *Danica McKellar*

When I (Dave) was attending prep school in New England, my physics professor designed the hardest exams possible, used a slide rule to compute the square root of each test score, then multiplied that score by ten. He was one of the sharpest people around, and just loved to stretch his mind, and the minds of his students, too. His goal was not so much to teach us Newton's Laws, but to teach us how to think about Newton's Laws.[1]

Most of us want to improve our thinking skills. The ability to think clearly, intelligently, and rapidly is one of our greatest resources and helps us to live a successful, abundant life. We were first allowed glimpses into the miraculous human brain with the invention of advanced brain scanning techniques. This knowledge has overturned much of our prior understanding about the way humans think. It is now accepted that every brain is unique, reflecting that individual's previous experience and education. In other words we each have the opportunity to build a better brain, day-by-day.

To build the best brain possible, we need to think like the coach of a football team, since there are eleven ways of thinking. All of these thinking abilities are involved in our everyday decisions and actions, which often engage several areas of our brain at once. This neurological workout continually forges new pathways and strengthens old ones.

The thinking team players are as follows (in order from basic to complex):[2]

Basic Level Thinking
Visual
Numerical
Recollective
Empathetic
Verbal
Predictive
Ethical
Creative
Critical
Reflective
Applied
Higher Order Thinking

Activities that work these different areas of our brain are known as "metacognitive" activities and actually strengthen our "thinking cap," the frontal cerebral cortex or learning center. When we engage in brain-jogging activities our frontal cerebral cortex is thickened, much the same way working with weights will strengthen arm muscles.

Our amazing brain has an automatic pilot gear (the one we

use while driving home engrossed in our music or while sleeping at night) but the metacognitive thinking powerhouse must be *requested*. For example, when we consider why we acted in a certain way, we are using *reflective thinking* skills that pull us from the past, through the present, and propel us into the future. Weakened reflective thinking can cripple our problem-solving abilities.

After following 10,000 children for fifteen years, Professor Michael Shayer at King's College in London found that some of the cognitive abilities of eleven- and twelve-year-olds had deteriorated on the average of two to three years compared to fifteen years earlier. The opposite was expected. Shayer speculated that the decline was because many learning activities important in elementary and secondary schools had fallen by the wayside. Art, music, and physical education had been cut from curriculums. He also suggested that creative thinking had, in too many cases, been replaced by overuse of technology (TV, video games, and calculators).[3]

Clear scientific thinking so desperately needed during those challenging academic years depends upon a well-functioning brain. A case can be made that "Use it or lose it" applies here. For instance, *numerical thinking* enhances logic and reasoning, while improving IQ and creating extra cognitive reserve. Such a reserve is a great nest egg to have if disease or brain injury strikes in the future.

My son, Christopher, to whom I dedicated my bestselling book *If God is So Good, Why Do I Hurt So Bad?*, is an inspiring example of the degree to which a brain injury can be overcome with courage, patience, and persistence. Christopher could read *The New York Times* by the time he was three, due in part to his interaction with the word games and other games available via the recently introduced Commodore 64.

But when he was six, about to go to first grade, he experienced a metabolic brain injury (like the one that had taken the life of his older brother), as a result of which he temporarily lost all the functions controlled by the areas of his brain that were affected—speech, movement, bodily functions.

But he still knew how to play the Commodore 64, and refused to give up, and thanks to the dogged determination of his mother who also refused to give up, he gradually recovered to the point where he could play that game again, using a magic marker taped in his hand as a way to punch the keys. Today he can type fifty words a minute. He graduated high school with his own peers, then graduated from college and even added a specialty associate's degree to his résumé.

Sometimes when I think of giving up, I think of Chris and all he has overcome. While none of us will ever know why our family was affected by this genetic deficiency, we do know that Chris accomplished more in a few years than just about anyone we've heard of because he never gave up, but instead recaptured what he could and built on that. I'm proud of him, and always will be.

SHARPER BRAIN TIPS

- When you're traveling, use a map instead of a GPS.
- Make your mind work harder whenever you have a choice.
- Read books rather than watching movies made from books.
- As you drive, listen to mind-sharpening audio instead of mind-numbing radio.
- Take a real tour of a local museum instead of a virtual tour of the Louvre. Better, take both tours.
- Create something from scratch instead of buying it premade, whether it is a pot pie or a potholder.
- For one week, do your math by hand, using a calculator only to check your results.
- Get an abacus and learn how to use it.
- If you ever have to figure out the square root of something, drag out and dust out that old slide rule and resurrect some synapses.

7

Just Dance

There are short-cuts to happiness, and dancing is one of them. *– Vicki Baum*

From a brain health perspective, dancing is a great activity. It can provide vigorous exercise, which by itself is one strategy for promoting brain health and cognition.[1] And learning new dance steps requires a type of learning known as learning for recall, which is important for brain health. Dancing is also a very social activity.

Exercise and fitness can improve brain function. For example, in a three-year study of forty-two healthy and active seniors, a group that engaged in Tai Chi was compared with a healthy and active control group of non-Tai Chi practitioners. The Tai Chi group demonstrated significantly better eye-hand coordination skills, measured in numerous ways.[2] The memorization and execution of forms (a continuous series of controlled, usually slow movements), which is central to Tai Chi, may be the source of this benefit.

Helen is in her late seventies. Years ago she joined a seniors group for dancing. They meet every week at the local synagogue and dance for ninety minutes with rehydration breaks. In her dancing group, they do mostly line dancing, because many come unaccompanied. They learn a new dance every couple of weeks. There is a mix of dances, because the dancers are not all of equal health, balance, or vitality. Many of the dances are quite vigorous. She only sits down when the dance has become too vigorous and there has been a lot of turning and spinning. She proudly says that she almost never sits down.

Dr. Majid Fotuhi, chairman of the Neurology Institute for Brain Health and Fitness and a neurology professor at Johns Hopkins University School of Medicine has mastered the tango. Fotuhi sees dancing as the perfect activity to keep his brain young. Sometimes people who want to delay or prevent late-life Alzheimer's ask Fotuhi, "What's the one thing I can do?" When that happens, he says, "Dance." He sees ballroom dancing as the perfect midlife lifestyle change because it combines physical activity, social interaction, and a mental challenge—remembering the steps![3]

Recent research indicates that the brain benefits from just observing dance nearly as much as from the physical experience of dancing itself. "Participants were trained for five consecutive days on dance sequences that were set to music videos in a popular video game context. They spent half of daily training physically rehearsing one set of sequences, and the other half passively watching a different set of sequences. Participants were scanned with functional magnetic resonance imaging (fMRI) prior to, and immediately following, the week of training. Viewing dance sequences that were only watched (and not danced) also was associated with significant activity in the brain's premotor areas, inferior parietal lobule, and basal ganglia [areas of the brain related to things like interpretation of sensory information, co-ordinated physical movement, and memory]."[4]

So whatever dance you like, from Acro dance to Zumba, don't

be bashful. Get out there and do it, and bring your brain along. Or watch someone else dancing. Your brain will benefit, either way.

But be forewarned—the energy and coordination of some forms of dancing can be extraordinary, so even watching can provide a workout. For example, every time I (Dave) watch the riverdancing presented in Michael Flatley's DVD *Feet of Flames*, my brain explodes, and it takes me about an hour to catch my breath!

SHARPER BRAIN TIPS

- Dance as an expression of rejoicing or celebration or worship. These types of dances are as old as humanity, often occurring in the form of what might be called "folk dancing." Some were celebrations of the hunt, but that would require a bow and arrows or big club, a loin cloth, and a roaring campfire.

- Watch dancing competitions that you consider wholesome on TV or via DVD.

- If you like ballroom dancing, you can dance by proxy as you watch one of the ten movies featuring Fred Astaire and Ginger Rogers. As they dance on your screen, imagine yourself to be either Fred or Ginger, and try not to get dizzy.

- If you can dance, be thankful that you can still move, since many who wish to dance can't do so any more.

- Find the nearest Aqua Zumba class, and give it a try!

8

Get Engaged

Your brain needs three things: oxygen, glucose, relationships.
– Dr. Henry Cloud

RESEARCHERS HAVE KNOWN FOR MANY YEARS THAT HAVING good social networks is good for your physical, mental, emotional, and spiritual well-being. But recent studies have found that supportive relationships can be advantageous to your brain health as well. The amount of contact you have with others is a good indication as to how well you will maintain sharp mental capabilities as you age.

AARP reports, "A major public-health study involving more than 116,000 participants found that people with strong relationships had less mental decline and lived more active, pain-free lives without physical limitations. Other studies suggest that people with the most limited social connections are twice as likely to die over a given period than those with the widest social networks. Many experts believe that social isolation may create a chronically stressful condition that accelerates aging."[1]

Loners don't age as well as those who keep socially active. Michael Merzenich, PhD, a neurobiologist at the University of

California, San Francisco, said, "As soon as you become captive in your room or your chair, you've got a problem. You become removed from the possibilities for excitement, for learning, and for engaging your brain with fun and surprise. Your brain needs you to get out and have those 1,000 daily surprises."[2]

Studies show that over the last several decades there has been an increase in social isolation in America. This is, in part, due to long work hours and hours spent using electronic gadgets from computers to tablets to cell phones to smart watches, versus spending at least some of that time with friends, in person. It is also related to the increased mobility of Americans due to job change and other factors, which make it difficult to maintain relationships and to develop new ones.

Older people often lead solitary lives because family and friends are no longer living close by. More and more people are opting to retire in a warmer climate, which often means leaving close relationships behind. Older adults also face the loss of marriage partners and other close relationships through death. There is a general decline in overall health, especially in older adults, after the death of a life partner. It is especially important for this age group to maintain and develop relationships and activities that help keep them connected, mentally alert, and physically healthy. This is easier for them if they are involved in senior centers, church groups, or other community organizations that provide opportunities for meaningful and active lifestyles.

Identifying opportunities for socialization in your community and combining that with your own innate talents can foster an enriched environment for your brain health. Research suggests a potentially important health role for maintaining socialization at any age. The activities you engage in throughout your life may have an impact upon your brain health and perhaps affect your vulnerability to neurodegenerative disease.

Social engagement challenges you to communicate effectively and to participate in complex social interactions. Social engagement fosters a dynamic, novel environment. It also requires a commitment to community and family that may promote a sense of belonging and purpose. The social network fostered by your social engagement can be helpful in many ways, including providing emotional support in times of distress.

Developing and sustaining relationships is one proactive, health-promoting activity that anyone can do. Margaret is eighty-five, living on her own after the death of her husband of fifty-nine years. She has chosen to remain in her own home because financially that makes the best sense. "After Bob died, I stayed by myself a lot and didn't really see anyone unless they came to see me," she said. "However, I found that my mental sharpness was slipping in small ways, such as forgetting to turn off the oven, and I realized that I needed to be around other people and get out more. I make sure that I spend time with friends at least once a week and stay connected by telephone. This has helped keep me alert. I also plan on joining a senior's Bible study."

SHARPER BRAIN TIPS

- Pursue social activities—join a club, take a class, join a gym, get involved in your community or church.
- Develop a hobby that involves you with others.
- Travel with friends.
- Take a class: golf, tennis, cooking, archery, photography, gardening, birdwatching, painting.
- Cultivate the friendships you have.
- Reduce relationships with people who tend to focus on negativity, gossip, and self-absorption.
- Attend reunions or other such gatherings.
- Form your own group if you can't find anything already organized related to your interests.
- Volunteer. It's one of the best ways to make new friends.

9

Stop Killing Yourself Slowly

Don't dig your grave with knife and fork.
– Old English Proverb

UNHEALTHY FOODS CAN HIJACK YOUR BRAIN IN TWO WAYS. They can harm you in the same manner that nicotine robs your neurons by clogging arteries and restricting blood flow. This reduces the levels of oxygen and healthy nutrients reaching your neurotransmitters. Or, unhealthy foods can cause a roller coaster or crash and burn effect in our body. These foods not only harm the brain but also can cause wild mood swings and unproductive behavior as well as obesity.

Dr. David Kessler, former FDA chief, calls the "culprit foods 'layered and loaded' with combinations of fat, sugar, and salt—and often so processed that you don't even have to chew much."[1] Neuroscientists continue to report that foods laden with fat/sugar combinations turn on the brain's dopamine pathway. This area is the pleasure center of the brain and is the very same place that fuels people's addiction to alcohol or drugs. It has even been reported recently that saturated bad fats can be a causative factor in Alzheimer's disease by damaging the blood vessel lining of the brain just as it does in the heart.[2] Additionally, an increasing number of neuroscientists believe that the wide variety of "neurotoxins" in our environment and our food are having a detrimental effect on health in general and brain health in particular. The list of these toxic substances is long, but includes certain artificial sweeteners and monosodium glutamate, a common food additive.[3]

Dr. Kessler has gathered researchers to find reasons why some people have such a hard time eating a healthy diet. He calls those who have great difficulty controlling what they eat "conditioned hyper eaters." Dr. Kessler found in a major study that this population of people report feeling a loss of control over food, and are preoccupied by food. He estimates that up to seventy million people have some degree of conditioned hyper eating.[4] Dr. Kessler's book, *The End of Overeating*, explains his strategies to overcome these brain and body damaging tendencies.

Many of these seventy million people carry a larger than normal amount of belly fat, which has been directly connected with brain shrinkage in old age.[5]

A more recent study found a possible explanation—your liver uses a certain protein (PPAR-alpha) to burn belly fat as the hippocampus in your brain uses to process memory. In people with a large amount of belly fat, the liver has to work overtime to try to metabolize that fat, and once this particular protein is used up in the liver, that organ "steals" it from the rest of your body, including your brain, in effect starving the hippocampus.[6]

As dangerous as saturated fat is in our food, sugary treats vie for first place among brain-damaging assassins. Dr. Larry McCleary has long been prodding us to eat healthy for the sake of our body and brain. He explains the stealth method that sugar and processed flour use to rob us of brainpower.

Dr. McCleary refers to the balance our bodies seek, by design, as the "Goldilocks Principle," named after the children's story of Goldilocks and the Three Bears in which Goldilocks is looking for things to be "just right" and does not want her porridge too hot or too cold, or her bed too soft or too hard. Dr. McCleary states that "neurons have similar needs when it comes to glucose and insulin levels . . . the major fuel the brain burns is sugar, or more precisely glucose."[7]

Good sugars (glucose), like good fats, are vital to the functioning of our brain, and the brain grabs onto 20 percent of the carbohydrates that we consume. Problems arise when we ingest sugar and simple carbohydrates in the wrong amounts and at the wrong times. If the timing and content are off we drag our body and brain onto a roller coaster for a wild ride throughout the day.

Bad brain foods cause our blood sugar levels to shoot up temporarily, which puts stress on the pancreas and triggers a powerful rush of insulin released into our bloodstream. This overabundance of insulin leads to plummeting blood sugar levels along with release of hormones manufactured in the adrenal glands, cortisol and epinephrine. High levels of these hormones in turn have the potential to kill brain cells and stress the liver. This roller coaster effect causes us to shift from feeling happy and energetic while "high" on glucose to becoming sleepy, irritable, unfocused, or even agitated—not a good way to have a productive day! To protect themselves from these highs and lows, neurons and other cells eventually become resistant to the action of the insulin. This can lead to diabetes.

What your body and brain crave is a steady flow of just the right amount and type of fuel throughout the day to provide a consistent blood glucose level. Eating good brain foods will give your brain the boost it needs to keep your memory and neurotransmitters humming along at productive levels.

SHARPER BRAIN TIPS

- Eat Blueberries. Researchers have found that blueberries help protect the brain from oxidative stress and may reduce the effects of age-related conditions such as Alzheimer's disease or dementia. One cup per day is "what the doctor ordered."
- Like Wild salmon. Salmon are rich in Omega-3 essential fatty acids, which support brain function.
- Enjoy Some Avocados. Avocados are fatty fruits, but the fat is monounsaturated, supporting healthy blood flow, which lowers blood pressure, a factor in cognitive decline over time.
- Munch Whole grains. Oatmeal, whole-grain breads, and brown rice promote cardiovascular health, and what's good for your heart is good for your brain.
- Consume Some Legumes. Beans help stabilize blood sugar levels, in part because their fiber moderates the delivery of glucose, which the brain depends on for fuel.
- Sip Freshly Brewed Tea. Two to three cups a day of freshly brewed tea—hot or iced—contains a modest amount of caffeine which can boost brain power by enhancing memory, focus, and mood. Tea also has potent antioxidants, especially the class known as catechines, which promote healthy blood flow. Take care, however, not to overcaffeinate yourself.
- Savor Some Dark Chocolate, which has powerful health-enhancing properties, contains several natural stimulants that enhance focus and concentration, and affects the production of endorphins.
- Eat some nuts daily to avoid going squirrelly over time. Almonds are the best all-round choice; one ounce daily (half a handful) is sufficient.

10

Play Furniture Roulette

The only difference between a rut and a grave is their dimensions. — Ellen Glasgow, author

It's easy to get into a rut, and we do it for many reasons: it saves time, we're too busy, life is too fast-paced, and keeping things the same is just easier. Most of us desire improvement, but we don't want to pay the price for it. But, did you know that making changes and getting out of your rut is good for your brain and will help you get more out of life?

People who lead mentally stimulating lives build a "cognitive reserve" in their brains. Some scientists suggest that stimulating the brain generates new neurons ("neurogenesis") and strengthens connections that already exist, which produces better brain performance and may lower the risk of developing Alzheimer's.[1] Others are studying neurogenesis using stem cells implanted in laboratory animals, with promising results.[2]

The key to establishing a "cognitive reserve" is leading a healthy, active lifestyle and stimulating the brain with learning and doing new things. Making changes "alters motor pathways in the brain and encourages new cell growth," according to Barbara E. Riley, director of the Ohio Department of Aging.[3] Besides being good for your brain health, it just makes life more interesting.

One of the easiest ways to get out of your "rut" is to change your living space. Even such simple things as planting new flowers in your yard, redecorating your kitchen, moving your furniture around, buying different color towels for the bathroom, and so on, will help stimulate those brain cells.

According to the Chinese, the goal in arranging (or rearranging) your living space, besides stimulating those brain cells, is to maximize feelings of safety and comfort, which will in turn positively affect your health, attitude, even your sense of success.[4] Creating a pleasing visual space in your home by the way you have things arranged is good for your physical, emotional, and spiritual health.

How do you get started? Go room by room in your home and take inventory. Here are some questions to watch for:

- Is the furniture arranged to maximize comfort, ease of movement, and to facilitate conversation and relationships with family and friends? Is your home office organized in a way to make your work easier? Is your kitchen arranged in a way that makes preparing a meal more of a pleasure than a chore?
- Is your color scheme soothing and pleasing to the eye? Do you have a variety of colors, or are your rooms monotone and perhaps boring?
- What about adding plants, pictures, or other decorative elements, and some interesting books with brightly colored jackets on your tables and shelves? Tired of those towels in the bathroom? Changing them can change the whole feel of the room.
- Would changing the lighting in some rooms help? Are there dark areas of your house, especially in the winter

that could use some better lighting? Are your curtains or window treatments blocking otherwise pleasant light from the outdoors?
- And, finally, does your home feel cluttered? If so, dispose of what you don't need, find new places for what you want to keep, and get everything more organized. If this step seems too daunting, imagine you are moving into a new home—about the size of this one—and you need to decide what to take and what to give away. Your mood and attitude may improve greatly as you simplify, room by room. And you may find some long-lost item as you tidy up—hopefully, it won't be alive!

SHARPER BRAIN TIPS

- Try taking a different route to any store you visit. Use some side roads and see if you can still find your way home without the GPS.
- Have lunch at 1 p.m. instead of precisely at noon. Have supper at 7 p.m. and pretend you're in France. Dialogue over dinner in French, if possible.
- Play a board game after supper instead of settling in front of the TV for the evening.
- Play yourself in chess.
- Take the cat or the goldfish for a walk—the latter if you can identify with the main character in the movie, *What About Bob?*
- Try an international restaurant next time you go out to eat. Make it an adventure.
- If your religious experience or personal faith is in a rut, renewing it could change your life from the inside-out, because personal faith is dynamic and active, like God's love for you: "GOD's loyal love couldn't have run out, his merciful love couldn't have dried up. They're created *new every morning*. How great your faithfulness!" (Lamentations 3: 22-23, MSG, emphasis added.)
- Don't try to change too many things at once. Habits take a lifetime to develop . . . or to change.

11

A Concert State of Mind

The brain needs a healthy soul and the soul needs a brain that works right.   *– Dr. Daniel Amen[1]*

IF YOU HAVE SPENT ANY AMOUNT OF TIME TALKING TO GOD AND encouraging others to do likewise, you need no convincing that meditation and prayer are good for us. In recent years, science is beginning to catch up to what we already know about this subject, in part due to high-tech scanning procedures that can capture images of the living brain at work and play. These technologies are showing that prayer and meditation alter the brain in ways that promote physical, emotional, cognitive, and relational health.

   Meditation, sometimes called "mindfulness," produces well-being and emotional balance by sculpting the brain, according to Dr. Daniel Amen. He describes meditation as a "concert state" for your brain. "By concert state I mean a relaxed body with a sharp, clear mind, much as you would experience at an exhilarating symphony. Achieving this state requires the ability to relax and focus."[1] A quick scan of the Bible produces twenty references about the practice of meditation, plus many more about prayer.

In *How God Changes Your Brain*, Dr. Andrew Newberg and Mark Robert Waldman illustrate how spiritual practices like intense prayer and/or meditation improve memory, cognition, and compassion while suppressing undesirable responses like anger, depression, and anxiety. They explain how these practices work directly on the brain circuits. For instance, the anterior cingulate in the brain is identified as our "neurological heart" and provides communication between the frontal lobe (thoughts and behavior) and the limbic system (feelings and emotions). The more active our anterior cingulate, the more empathy we will have and the less likely we will be to react with fear and anger.[2]

Gus was a participant in one of Newberg and Waldman's studies on the benefits of meditation. He had come to the clinic because of concerns about his faltering brain, but had never meditated a day in his life. He overcame his skepticism and was determined to give it a try. He was prescribed a routine of twelve minutes of mindfulness exercises a day. "After only eight weeks of practice his brain was scanned and showed remarkable increase of neural activity in the prefrontal cortex, an area involved in helping to maintain a clear, focused attention upon a task."[3]

Intense prayer has similar effects upon our brain. People who make prayer a part of their regular routine actually train and modify their brain in a way that is believed to be permanent. The more one believes in what he or she is praying about, the stronger the response will be. Roman Catholic nuns who had practiced "centering prayer" on a regular basis for a minimum of fifteen years were studied. The goal of centering prayer is to get in touch with the heart of God, which brings about a sense of peace, comfort, and compassion. The brain scans found that this kind of intense prayer brought about significant positive long-term neurological changes.[4] Perhaps this is because prayer has a way of fixing our mind on our Maker, who is like Polaris, never moving. Our overall sense of well-being can be enhanced, and our anxieties and stress can be reduced because we know that he is always there for us.

Numerous studies have verified that we begin to form a mental image of God when we are just little children. This might begin, for example, on our very first Christmas when we are surrounded with all kinds of visual, auditory, and olfactory stimuli, which we connect with Jesus' birthday. Since, as young children, we think in pictures and cannot as yet form abstract thoughts, our view of God and Jesus is formed by what we experience and what we hear the adults around us saying. The whole experience of reading the Christmas story, setting up a nativity scene, making special cookies, the arrival of grandparents laden with gifts, the beautiful tree, and the singing of carols all form positive images of a loving God.

This early view continues to evolve as we age and have additional positive experiences related to the character of God. Studies have shown that if a person was exposed to God or Jesus as a young child, a memory circuit is established and is triggered each time the person has similar experiences or even just thinks about God. As a result, prayer or meditation that centers on a loving God taps into and strengthens early neuronal pathways, paving the way toward a more "adult" experience of security and serenity even when experiencing times of distress.

SHARPER BRAIN TIPS

- Set aside part of your home for prayer and meditation.
- Establish a place where you can sit or kneel.
- If you wish, include items with special meaning to you aimed at establishing a worshipful environment for your body, mind, and spirit.
- Engage in these devotional exercises regularly and at an established time. Early morning works best for most.[5]
- Stay in tune with your Maker, and your concert state of mind will become a concert way of life.

12

Stoke Your Belly Fire

The brain wants to learn. It wants to be engaged as a learning machine.   – Dr. Michael Merzenich

YOU MAY HAVE LEARNED IN SCHOOL THAT THE NUMBER OF brain cells you have is fixed. With this in mind, educators encouraged us to act with care to preserve whatever number of brain cells we already had. At the same time, this teaching may have created a sense of futility that our brainpower was fixed and that, as we aged, the best we could do was to limit our losses.

Today we know that the brain is very capable of growth even into our senior years.[1] And there is even more good news. Cognitive performance in older adults appears to be improving over time. A study with a US and UK sample found that older people today show less cognitive impairment than earlier cohorts. Because of improvements in medicine, health care, and other social factors, many people do perform well in old age and continue to learn new skills.[2] One key to retaining brain health into our later years seems to be to keep learning. Learning stimulates the brain. To date, no particular regimen of learning has been shown to be better than another, so feel free to pursue that life-long passion. Commit your brain to learning what is fun and satisfying.

Our friend Bruce Incze told us, "My father immigrated to this country in 1951. He was a poor war refugee who brought with him his twelve-pound, 1937 Remington Junior typewriter, equipped with Hungarian as well as English characters. Dad was a writer. His typewriter is now an heirloom and still works. Being a passionate writer and a practical man, at 65 years of age, he realized that learning to word process on a computer would benefit his writing endeavors. Thus, his passion (writing) and a need for learning (word processing) were combined. Learning to operate a computer was slow and frustrating at first, but the brain did not object to the workout.

"At 69 years of age, Dad was awarded the Gold Medal for *Footprints of Destiny Lane*[3] by the Árpád Academy of Arts and Sciences, a society for the preservation of Hungarian culture. After that, he learned one operating system after another. He even had to abandon his favorite word processing software as it became obsolete. This was somewhat traumatic as no other word processing program supports the ease of bilingual writing he had come to master.

"Given this new obstacle, why persevere? Because he still had a fire in his belly to write. Through the years, he published many non-commercial books. Even in his early 90s, he continued to learn new computer technologies. (He was intentional to say, 'I am 94 years of age' and not 'I am 94 years old.') He had moments of frustration, but he learned new skills because they were needed to express his passion through writing. Until he died at age 97, he remained as sharp as a tack and a delight to engage in conversation. And even in his final year, he spent hours a day on his writing projects."

Your brain is a resilient organ. Even if you have allowed yourself to become something of a couch potato, it is never too late to try something new. The largest controlled clinical trial to date found that memory, concentration, and problem-solving skills of healthy adults ages sixty-five and older were improved by cognitive training.[4]

In his book, Spark, John J. Ratey, MD, describes the importance of challenging your mind at any age. "It's no coincidence that study after study shows that the more education you have, the more likely you are to hang onto your cognitive abilities and stave off dementia," Raley says. "But it's not necessarily about the diploma. It's just that those who have spent a lot of time in school are more likely to remain interested in learning. . . . Novel experiences demand more from your brain, and this builds its ability to compensate. You get more . . . connections, more neurons, and more possibilities."[5]

Dave's friend Len has been "retired" for some time, but he has kept his brain sharp by immersing himself continually in new hobby-type engagements, including building a huge model train layout to scale, building ships to scale in a bottle, tackling extremely detailed woodwork, and learning digital photography and photo editing. Len never seems to tire of trying new things.

Remember, you're never too old to try something new, or to find a new way to do something "old." Your choice. Are you going to be 100 years old, or 100 years of age? The former is counting down; the latter is counting up. Isn't it about time to erase this phrase from your vocabulary: "I'm too old to. . . ."

SHARPER BRAIN TIPS

- Enroll in a course at your local community college—in something you know nothing about.
- Adopt projects that require learning new skills; for example, refurbish a boat or automobile, learn to knit, spin, or how to make quilts.
- Join a club focused on strategic games: chess, bridge, "Settlers of Catan," "Carcassonne," etc.
- If you like to cook, try new recipes; further, adjust those recipes to your own needs and tastes. Share them with others; perhaps even publish them online.

13

How Do You Want Your Change?

Nothing so needs reforming as other people's habits.
– Mark Twain

THE OLDER WE GET, THE HARDER IT IS TO CHANGE OUR habits, partly because it is so difficult to change our way of thinking, and how we think controls what we do. Quite often, it isn't that we don't *want* to change, especially when it is easy to see that a change one way or another might be really good for us. Yet sometimes, even knowing that a return to an old habit will most likely result in severe consequences is still not enough motivation to prevent the continuing practice of that particular habit.

It's not just a matter of choice, or everyone who wants to amend their bad habits could "just say no" to them and "yes" to something else. For example, anyone for whom overeating is a problem could just say "no" to unhealthy food, and "yes" to healthy food. And there wouldn't be so many trying-to-recover alcoholics falling off the wagon when six month's sobriety would give them a chance of a liver transplant and extended life. Willpower alone is not enough to effect lasting habit change because this kind of personal revamping requires changing your habits of *thought*, which ultimately can affect the power of your *will*.

Phillip, a Christian doctor just out of his residency program, wanted to provide a good life for his family. So he joined a lucrative practice of excellent doctors believing he could serve his patients and give his family what they needed to have a wonderful life. He soon discovered there was a list of "unspoken" expectations that went with the job. It was strongly advised that he buy a house in the "right" part of town and send his children to the best private school. In addition, there were many social activities that were expected in order to be a "solid part of the community." This all sounded reasonable to Phillip and his wife, who set about conforming to the lifestyle that was presented and modeled by the senior doctors in the group.

The first year was great. They loved their beautiful new home, convincing themselves that the stretch on their budget was worth it. The children seemed to be thriving in their private school. As their busy social life took more and more of their time, they began to make excuses for why they had to miss church-related activities. Phillip reasoned that a doctor has very limited free time and it is important to the practice to fulfill one's social obligations, which did not seem to include accepting invitations to social events or his former "religious" friends, who ultimately stopped asking.

Phillip was working longer and longer hours, but always felt he was behind schedule. He could not relax and wasn't sleeping well. One of his children began having serious behavioral problems and his wife was having severe headaches. Phillip talked to a trusted pastor, who helped him see that the "rewards" he was receiving for his hard work and striving were not producing results consistent with the values and goals that he had espoused when he had started practice. Instead, he had gradually accepted another way of thinking and the habits of thought that came with it. As a result he had slowly transformed into a person he hardly recognized, and his entire self—body, mind, spirit, and relationships—was suffering.

"Doctors aren't the only ones who get caught in this trap," the pastor explained. "Pastors do, too. In fact, anybody can. The apostle Paul described this conflict in Romans 7, and I like to picture it as a see-saw, with one seat being your mind and the other seat your emotions, and the fulcrum, upon which the board pivots, your will. Your mind and emotions move the board, easily or with more difficulty, depending on where you focus your will. In this case, you want your mind to move your emotions, using your will for leverage."

Phillip realized that he had allowed his emotions and the connections that they offered—status, self-satisfaction, happiness, security—to hijack the goal that mattered most to him, to be a faithful follower of Christ, whom the doctor knew to be the only source of life to the full. It was time for a change, starting with his emotional reaction to the "cues" that he had allowed to attach themselves to counterfeits.

For example, one day as he drove home in his Mercedes, he countered the false pride he often connected to that luxurious car with this thought: I don't need a Mercedes, when a Ford will do to get to work and back. And, when he walked into his beautiful, spacious, impeccably landscaped home that night, his first thought was: We don't need a home this extravagant. We'll downsize as soon as possible. This was the start of a new life for Phillip and his family.[1]

Matching our behavior to our goals is governed by the "executive center" located in the prefrontal cortex of the brain, which is constantly bombarded with the promise of rewards for behavior—buy this, be cool; use this, be like Mike. These rewards are often connected with visual cues, called logos, which is why so many people are willing to pay for clothing with company logos prominently displayed. And for people of means, visual cues often come with a big price tag and a little hood ornament.

You can change your habits. Actually, it's more like an exchange of habits, replacing unhealthy ones with those that are healthier. The change begins in your mind, which can control your emotions and even change them, putting your will to work as you will God's will. The apostle Paul wrote, just a few verses later than where he described the conflict just discussed, "Do not be conformed to this world, but be transformed by the renewal of your mind, that by testing you may discern what is the will of God, what is good and acceptable and perfect" (Romans 12:2, ESV).

SHARPER BRAIN TIPS

- Periodically review your current life goals to be sure they are aligned with healthy living.
- Pay careful attention to your thought patterns: Are they constructive or plagued by anxiety and guilt? Are they focused more on the cares and concerns of this present life, or on spiritual matters?
- Would you describe yourself as satisfied or restless? Which would you rather be?
- What visual clues do you find it hard to resist? How can you change this habitual reaction to a more constructive one?
- Can you identify with the conflict described by the apostle Paul in Romans 7:15-25? If so, can you find something in that passage that points toward a resolution to the conflict?
- Find an accountability partner and be on the lookout for unhealthy patterns of behavior (habits) that can lurk around the edges of your life space, waiting to gain a front row seat.
- Identify one "status" symbol in your life, and exchange it for what you think it's better than.

14

A Funny Thing Happened on the Way to the Foramen

If we couldn't laugh we would all go insane.

– Jimmy Buffet

Humor is good for you. As Solomon wrote, "A merry heart does good, like medicine" (Proverbs 17:22, NKJV). Our sense of humor reflects an often under-celebrated characteristic of our Creator, whose image we reflect. He laughs; we laugh, starting when we're babies. Laughing spans age, gender, language, and culture. It's good for your mind, body, spirit, and relationships. We make each other laugh and we respond to laughter in others. They laugh; we laugh. It's contagious.

Enter the punster with the question: Why don't cannibals eat clowns? Answer: Because they taste funny! This pun employs a word that has more than one meaning ("funny"), while mixing in a bit of ambiguity and absurdity. Perhaps you've heard it before. But it's less likely that you've imagined an article in a peer-reviewed professional journal (*The Journal of Neuroscience*) with the title: "Why Clowns Taste Funny: The Relationship between

Humor and Semantic Ambiguity."

The study, using a highly sensitive functional Magnetic Resonance Imaging (fMRI), demonstrated that humorous word twisting, as happens in punning, stimulates not just a loud guffaw, but a significant amount of activity in parts of your brain connected with higher levels of functioning. In other words, puns are brain candy. The more complicatedly ambiguous, the better. The researchers even included in their report the punny question: Why were the teacher's eyes crossed? Answer: Because she could not control her pupils.[1]

To summarize the study in lay terms, enjoying highly ambiguous and very funny jokes keeps your brain working like very few other things can. Just be careful, of course, not to laugh your head off.

Psychological benefits of laughter include:

- reduction of stress and anxiety,
- elevation of mood,
- increased coping skills,
- increased self-esteem.

Laughter helps combat depression. After all, it's hard to laugh and feel sad at the same time.

Physically, laughter boosts the immune system, lowers blood pressure, decreases stress hormones, decreases pain, and increases lung function, among other benefits. The physical act of laughing is important, so a heartfelt snicker simply won't do. The exertions involved in producing laughter increase oxygenation in general, while triggering an increase in endorphins, the opioid neurotransmitters known for their feel-good-effect.

"Social laughter" fosters closeness in a group. Dr. R. I. M. Dunbar and colleagues tested resistance to pain before and after bouts of social laughter through experiments using comedy videos. Participants wore frozen wine cooler sleeves or blood pressure cuffs while watching the videos. The results showed that laughing increased pain tolerance, whereas simply feeling good in a group setting did not.[2]

Neuroscientist Dr. Robert Provine studied laughter as it relates to couples. Uniquely human, laughter is, first and foremost, a social signal—it disappears when there is no audience, which may be as small as one other person—and it binds people together. It synchronizes the brains of speaker and listener so that they are emotionally attuned. Provine writes that, "Laughter establishes—or restores—a positive emotional climate and a sense of connection between two people, who take pleasure in the company of each other." Levity can defuse anger and anxiety, and therefore, can pave the path to intimacy. Provine states that, "laughter is not primarily about humor, but about social relationships."

Sources of humor are all around you and your laugh receptors are just waiting to be activated. One of the plusses of e-mail and social media is that often someone will send or post something that is just downright funny and you find yourself laughing so hard it hurts. This is wonderful, especially if you've been having a less than wonderful day.

Recently a friend pulled into a Starbucks drive-thru for a cup of coffee. She was absent-mindedly writing a song in her head and pulled too far forward—past the microphone where she was supposed to place her order. She stopped, rolled down the window and didn't realize she had rolled down the back window. Her dog in the back seat loved being able to look out the window. When she realized her mistake, she backed up to place her order and found the entire barista staff laughing. The staff told her that all they could see in their video camera was her dog with its head out the window eagerly waiting to place an order. They had never had a dog want to place an order before. The excited pooch received a puppy latte for starting the staff's Monday with a laugh. Arf! The woman expanded her enjoyment by posting the story on Facebook.

SHARPER BRAIN TIPS

- Figure out who or what makes you laugh and seek more of it.
- Learn to laugh at yourself. For example, you can either laugh or get depressed when you find your glasses in the freezer.
- Look for opportunities to share something funny with others. Social media sites are excellent for this.
- Learn some jokes and spring them on your friends and coworkers. For example, "Did you know that Noah's dog had a speech impediment?" "All it could say was 'Ark! Ark!'" Or try one of these: "I'm reading a book about anti-gravity. I can't put it down," or, "I used to think I was indecisive, but now I'm not so sure."
- Tell stories, like this true one about a guy at the airport, checking in at the gate, when an airport employee asked, "Has anyone put anything in your baggage without your knowledge?" To which the man replied, "If it was without my knowledge, how would I know?" The employee smiled knowingly and nodded, "That's why we ask."
- Quote humorous people, one of the best being Mark Twain, who warned: "Be careful about reading health books. You may die of a misprint."
- Oh, and before you turn the page, take another look at the title of this chapter. Did you read the final word as "forum" as in the title of that farcical 1960s Broadway play? Or did you read it "foramen," which is a part of your brain? It's just another example of a play on words. Get it?
- Join a pun-a-day Internet program. Here's one you might like: "This girl said she recognized me from the vegetarian club, but I'd never met herbivore."

15

Getting Your Marbles Back

> *... if you keep most of your marbles intact, you can add a note of wisdom to the coming generation.* – Clint Eastwood

Imagine that you are at your 50th high school class reunion, surrounded by people who seem older than you are, and you recognize their faces. But for the life of you, you can't recall the names of your three best friends who are chatting over in the corner. *What is this?* you wonder. *Sudden onset Alzheimer's? Is there such a thing?* As your anxiety increases, your ability to recall the names of others in the room decreases. *I need to get out of here before I embarrass myself*, you decide. *I feel like I'm losing my marbles.*

Marian felt something like this when she enlisted in a three-month memory enhancement program offered by the Neurology Institute for Brain Health and Fitness (NIBHF) in Lutherville, Maryland. At 78, she felt that her mental functioning was declining, and she was worried. Lately, her memory had been slipping and she'd had more "senior moments" than she could count. At the NIBHF, she learned about factors still within her control that would improve her cognitive abilities—including her diet, physical exercise, stress reduction techniques, getting more sleep, *and brain training.*

Dr. Majid Fotuhi, MD, PhD, and founder of the clinic, described his personal satisfaction with Marian's results, which included the fact that she had learned to memorize twenty things at a time, until by the end of her program, she had memorized 100 things. "By the time she returned to her family," Dr. Fotuhi said, "she could recite the complete list, backward and forward, and even start in the middle. For example, if we asked her for item number sixty-eight, she could name that and then go backward and forward from there. Our staff felt like we had introduced this woman to a new life! She had come in worried that she was losing it, and had gone back home able to impress her grandkids with her new skill."

Over the past few years, Fotuhi and others have been challenging age-old assumptions about old-age decline, which has been a subject of study and discussion since the 7th Century BC. The Greek philosopher Pythagoras described a "normal" cognitive slide that would begin "in one's 60s and, by one's 80s, would lead to the 'imbecility of infancy.'"[1]

This perspective was the major view, with some minor variations (for example, people with dementia were treated as witches in the Renaissance era) until as recently as 1907, when Alois Alzheimer described "plaques and tangles" in the brain of a young patient with progressive cognitive decline in his report, "About a peculiar disease of the cerebral cortex." For the next ninety years, much of the research into "Alzheimer's disease" (AD) focused on these amyloid plaques and tangles, with the dominant view becoming that these caused AD.[2]

The publication of the "Nun Study" (1997) forced researchers to focus more broadly, because the degree of cognitive impairment the nuns had shown before their deaths did not correlate well with the amount of tangles and plaques that were found in their brains post-mortem. In other words, many of the nuns had retained more clarity of thought and overall functioning than the amounts of tangles and plaques found should have allowed if those were the primary causes of AD.

It was time to step back and consider the causes of age-related cognitive decline more broadly, including the relatively new thought that it might be treatable (to slow it down) or even—who would dare suggest it?—reversible. In other words, it was time to challenge neuroscientists to change the way they think about thinking.

New imaging technology has made it possible to pinpoint and measure changes that occur in specific areas of the brain, the most important of which (in terms of short-term memory) is the hippocampus. Research has shown a correlation between the size of one's hippocampus and the risk of developing AD—the larger the hippocampus, the less the risk; the smaller the hippocampus, the greater likelihood of decline.

Since causes and cures related to AD include factors from vigorous exercise versus stagnation, proper nutrition versus the typical Western diet, learning relaxation methods and better sleep to offset stress, plus other concerns, the most effective cognitive improvement program will involve experts from all the disciplines in question.

"What we've done," Dr. Fotuhi explained, "is to identify twelve factors that can either grow or shrink your hippocampus. Our program educates participants about these factors, encouraging them to decrease practices that cause shrinkage, and to increase practices that cause growth. The hippocampus is constantly creating neurons [brain cells]. If they're put to use, they stick around and the size of the hippocampus increases. We can see that increase with before-and-after MRIs. If those cells are not used, they slough off like other cells in the body and are lost. With our program, we can prevent the loss of these cells and the results have been amazing."[3]

SHARPER BRAIN TIPS

- Get Moving: As little as three months of walking just three days a week results in a measurable growth in the hippocampus.
- De-stress: Eight weeks of stress reduction can lead to measurable growth in the hippocampus.
- Feed Your Brain: A healthy diet balanced with fruits, vegetables, grains, and dairy has been linked to better cognitive performance. Diets rich in the nutrients Vitamin E; Vitamin B12; folate, and DHA, available as supplements, have also been shown to aid in cognition.
- Manage Your Health Well: Diabetes, high cholesterol, high blood pressure, stroke, and obesity can all make your brain, and especially your hippocampus, smaller.
- Use It or Lose It. Brain cells, like muscles cells, thrive on stimulation and can readily grow in size.
- Sleep! Chronic sleep problems can cause the hippocampus to shrink. If you have trouble sleeping, you may have sleep apnea. Consult a reputable sleep center.
- Take your ease—daily, weekly, annually—or you may experience disease instead.

16

Brain Safe Your Home

Minds, like bodies, will often fall into a pimpled, ill-conditioned state from mere excess of comfort. – Charles Dickens

YOUR HOME MAY BE COZY, FULL OF TOYS, AND GOOD BOOKS. You might have DVD movies with a wide-screen TV. You might have a hot tub in which to unwind after a hard day at work, or a big kitchen in which to relax by preparing and cooking gourmet dinners. But your home may also be filled with safety and health hazards!

Have you ever inspected your home to see how many hazards you might find? Many injuries and illnesses occur in the home environment. These include head injuries from accidental falls, lead poisoning of children, and poisoning from inhaling or ingesting a variety of common substances—all of which can be prevented with common sense and good housekeeping. Use your good mind to protect your brain from injury!

Chemicals may be found throughout your home such as bleach, ammonia, roach traps, nail polish remover, isopropyl alcohol, drain cleaner, carpet cleaner, paints, paint thinners, gasoline, glues, and other adhesives. Serious consequences can result from exposure to pesticides and their residues, indoor toxicants, tobacco smoke, solvents, and combustion gases such as carbon monoxide. Read the labels of all the chemicals you store in and around your house. You may be surprised by what you find. Labels contain important information such as warnings to keep them out of reach of children. This does not mean you should get rid of all these chemicals. Rather, you should respect them for what they can do if they are not handled and stored properly.

Carbon monoxide is a very dangerous gas, partly because it is colorless and odorless—it is a silent killer.[1] Whenever a gas oven or heater or automobile is running in an enclosed space there can be danger from carbon monoxide poisoning. Early symptoms can include headache and dizziness. Carbon monoxide poisoning affects the heart, lungs, and brain. It interferes with the heart and brain's ability to get oxygen. Babies, infants, and the elderly are most vulnerable. But you can protect yourself by installing carbon monoxide detectors, which are similar in size to many smoke detectors, in your home.

According to the US Centers for Disease Control and Prevention, approximately 250,000 children aged one to five years have blood lead levels greater than the level at which action should be taken.[2] Lead poisoning can occur with no obvious symptoms or warning signs. However, children's blood lead levels can be checked. Lead poisoning is preventable. Lead-based paint and lead-contaminated dust are major sources of exposure even though lead-based paint was banned in 1978 in the US. Old homes deteriorate and the lead paint peels off and becomes dust around the house where children play. Children under the age of six years old are at greatest risk because of the effect of lead on their development. Other sources of lead include contaminated soil and toys, jewelry, cookware, and cosmetics that contain lead.

In your home, there may be other risks to children and adolescents, including access to electrical outlets (for young children), glues and other adhesives used in hobbies, alcohol that is made for consumption, prescription drugs that affect the brain, and even—hard to believe—your office supplies, including various adhesives, solvents, even "canned air."

Kyle's policeman father learned this the hardest way:

> On March first I left for work at 10 p.m. At 11 p.m. my wife went down and kissed Kyle goodnight. At 5:30 a.m. the next morning Kathy went downstairs to wake Kyle up for school, before she left for work. He was sitting up in bed with his legs crossed and his head leaning over. She called to him a few times to get up. He didn't move. He would sometimes tease her like this and pretend he fell back asleep. He was never easy to get up. She went in and shook his arm. He fell over. He was pale white and had the straw from the Dust Off can coming out of his mouth. He had the new can of Dust Off in his hands. Kyle was dead.
>
> I am a police officer and I had never heard of this. My wife is a nurse and she had never heard of this. We later found out from the coroner, after the autopsy, that only the propellant from the can of Dust Off was in his system. No other drugs. Kyle had died between midnight and 1 a.m.
>
> I found out that using Dust Off is being done mostly by kids ages nine through fifteen. They even have a name for it. It's called dusting. A takeoff from the Dust Off name. It gives them a slight high for about ten seconds. It makes them dizzy. A boy who lives down the street from us showed Kyle how to do this about a month before. Kyle showed his best friend. Told him it

was cool and it couldn't hurt you. It's just compressed air. It can't hurt you. . . .

Kyle was wrong.[3]

SHARPER BRAIN TIPS

- Check your home for harmful chemicals, paints, varnishes, insecticides, and bleach.
- Avoid exposure to carbon monoxide—add carbon monoxide detectors.
- Beware of lead exposure for children; electrical hazards for small children.
- Keep your prescription medication and supplements in a safe place: small children can ingest fatal doses of vitamins or other over-the-counter medications.
- Store office supplies that might be dangerous in a safe place.
- Apply the principles of "Universal Design," which include: equitable use, flexibility in use, simple and intuitive use, perceptible information, tolerance for error, low physical effort, size and space for approach and use. These guidelines help eliminate hazards for older adults.
- Each day, stand in the middle of one room in your home and ask yourself: "Is there anything here that is hazardous to a child . . . an adolescent . . . an older adult?" Take action as appropriate.

17

Eureka!

If you could use a video camera to watch the brain respond to experiences, I have no doubt you would see it growing, retracting, reshaping.
— Larry Squire, MD

FANTASTIC IMAGES OF THE BRAIN REVEALED BY HIGH-TECH scans amaze and delight researchers as they study the brain. Not only can they inspect the brain's anatomy closely, but they can also watch as different areas light up in brilliant colors as people engage in various activities. The old idea that our brain is a stagnant organ hidden away in our skull and slowly wearing out has given way to the belief that our brain grows new neuronal pathways in response to mental challenges. The process of discovery is one such invigorating challenge. And it brings an added benefit, too—the joy of finding something new.

Deep in our gray matter is an area with a catchy name, anterior cingulate cortex, which has been recently dubbed the "eureka circuits." This is where hundreds of neurons become active when we are in the process of exploring.

We've all had "aha" moments, which can materialize without warning when we change how we perceive a situation. Sometimes it's a solution to a gnarly problem; or it could be suddenly recognizing a face or even finally getting a joke! As simple as these discoveries may seem, they represent the culmination of intense and complex changes in the brain that require a lot more neural resources than ordinary analytical thinking.

Dr. Mark Wheeler, a psychologist at the University of Pittsburgh, was the first to map the decision-making and evidence-gathering process prior to the actual "eureka" moment. Using brain-scanning equipment, he found that our brain is highly engaged when our mind is wandering and is working quite hard right before this moment of insight.[1]

Researchers report that a serene mental state is fertile ground for eureka moments. Newton's discovery about gravity occurred in an orchard when he saw an apple fall from a tree. Descartes was in bed watching flies on his ceiling when the ideas foundational to "Cartesian coordinates" came to him. Archimedes was about to take a bath; when he stepped in, he noticed that the water level rose, and suddenly he realized that the volume of water displaced must equal the volume of the part of his body that was submerged. The implication was that the volume of irregular objects (such as one's leg) could be calculated with precision, a problem that previously had seemed unsolvable to scientists. Legend has it that Archimedes was so excited by his discovery that he leapt from the tub and then "streaked" through the streets of Syracuse, naked, shouting, "Eureka! I've got it."

All around us, we can see others experiencing the excitement and joy of discovery. Think of a child's Easter egg hunt. The child doesn't even have to be an "egg lover" to become totally involved in the challenge of the hunt. Each child is on high alert as he or she scrambles and climbs and dives for those hidden colored eggs! Treasure hunts have the same allure, even for adults, some of whom end up turning their avocation into a vocation.

Discovery's benefits are not limited to what it does for you;

you can also gain benefits by joining in the excitement of others as they make their own discoveries. One of the many joys of being a grandparent is getting a phone call from your grandchild describing their latest discovery. Our (Jim and Bobbie's) then five-year-old granddaughter had just moved to Florida when on one of her first trips to the beach she called, her voice full of excitement. "Nana, guess what I found? The ocean is full of baby seahorses!" she exclaimed, too thrilled to take a breath. "They are swimming all around and look just like real horses except they have a mermaid tail . . . and they don't even bite!" This day of discovery ushered in a great learning experience for all of us as we learned more about Florida marine life.

As Ralph Waldo Emerson said, "We are all inventors, sailing out on a voyage of discovery; guided by a private chart, of which there is no duplicate." So set sail into each new day with the expectation of discovering something. Reawaken the sense of wonder you had as a child, whether it was watching seahorses swim or watching a Monarch butterfly emerge from its cocoon. From armadillos to zebras, everything is wonder-full, in its own way. And it's inspiring to consider why the Creator made such a magnificent variety of creatures to live with us here. But remember, when you discover something new, keep your clothes on if you must run about shouting "Eureka!"

SHARPER BRAIN TIPS

- Recall something creative you loved doing as a child, and do it again.
- Visit far-away places. If you can't go in person, take a virtual tour of those places by computer.
- Read an adventure book. Be the main character.
- Compile an album of close-up photos of all the flowers within 100 yards of your front door.
- Select something in your home that you use and enjoy regularly. Try to invent something that will improve it.

18

Feed Your Gold Mind

Brain cells continually produce new dendrites and receptors, grow new synapses . . . and alter the essence of the neurotransmitter soup that stimulates brain activity.

– Jean Carper

WE HAVE A "GOLD MIND" AT OUR DISPOSAL IN THE FORM of the more than fifty neurotransmitters that surge through our brain every moment of every day. These neurotransmitters have exotic names, including: serotonin, norepinephrine, dopamine, and GABA (gamma-aminobutyric acid).

Neurotransmitters are chemical messengers stored in tiny packets located throughout the brain and gastrointestinal tract that enable neurons to communicate with one another. When a neurotransmitter is released it flashes across the junction or synapse at the end of one brain cell onto the receptor of another. Since each neuron can have multiple synapses, it has the ability to communicate with literally thousands of other neurons each microsecond! This amazing ability enables us to maintain positive moods and attitudes. The health of our neurotransmitter system also affects such important functions as memory, intelligence, and creativity.

Researchers at MIT discovered a key player in the complex chain of events controlling the release of our neurotransmitters from neuron to neuron. Tiny proteins, called complexins, are the gatekeepers. "The neurotransmitters are like racehorses. They chomp at the bit until they get the signal to dash toward the finish line . . . complexins are the gatekeepers that prevent the neurotransmitters from releasing prematurely."[1]

Neurotransmitters are so vital to keeping traffic moving on our biochemical highway that without them our brain would instantly cease to function. Not one message could be sent or received, and the power would go out. Because these messengers are so vital to *who we are*, scientists have been relentless in studying ways to protect and strengthen them. Genetics play a part, and some of us inherit lower levels of certain neurotransmitters; others have depleted amounts due to overwhelming stressful life experiences. When the makeup of our neurotransmitters is out of balance, depression and its companions take over. When needed, anti-depressants can help to balance our neurotransmitter levels and improve our symptoms. Other, non-pharmaceutical approaches may help also including counseling, exercise, improvement in relationships, practicing your faith, and better nutrition.

Years ago, Dr. Richard Wurtman of MIT suggested that one's diet contributes significantly to the types of neurotransmitters our body makes and how they travel about. Many people were incredulous. Since then, it has become accepted that the seat of our emotions, the limbic system, needs certain nutrients in order to function properly. Good fats, like Omega-3 fatty acids found in fish, are important. A well-rounded diet that includes a reasonable amount of protein and a wide variety of whole food nutrients, including green leafy plants, is essential to maintaining brain health. Proteins are the building blocks of neurotransmitters and are crucial to balancing levels of dopamine and serotonin, for instance. It is safe to say that eating a healthy, varied diet helps to support our "gold mind" day by day. That's why feeding our brain well is crucial to maintaining optimal health.

> **SHARPER BRAIN TIPS**
>
> - View your neurotransmitters as a gold mine.
> - Do all you can to protect them.
> - Provide them a balanced and nutritious diet—we're using "diet" here in its root meaning of one's daily routine.
> - Exercise regularly to enhance blood flow to your brain.
> - If you suffer with depression, be thankful there are treatments that can help your neurotransmitters recover . . . and do not hesitate to seek that help.
> - Choose slow food over fast food.

19

Don't Eat Squirrel Brains

In our family, we saw it as a prized piece of meat, and if he [Dad] shared it with you, you were pretty happy. Not that he was stingy, but there's just not much of a squirrel brain.
— Janet Norris Gates[1]

SQUIRREL BRAINS ARE A BACKWOODS SOUTHERN DELICACY, especially in Kentucky, where the gray squirrel has been the state's official wild game animal since 1968, with an annual harvest estimated at 1.5 million critters a.k.a. *sciurus carolinensis*. In some rural areas the predilection for this particular treat owes itself to tradition as well as to taste.

Kentucky physicians Drs. Erick Weisman and Joseph Berger noticed that in a period of just four years, eleven cases of a human form of transmissible spongiform encephalopathy, called Creutzfeldt-Jakob disease [similar to mad cow disease], had been diagnosed in rural western Kentucky. All the patients were squirrel-brain eaters; thus, the new disease name "mad squirrel disease."[2]

Eating brains or any parts of the central nervous system of any animal is somewhat risky. Despite this, the brains of pigs, horses, cattle, monkeys, chickens, and goats are consumed with gusto in some parts of the world. Since the first outbreak of Mad Cow Disease, mad cows have been identified in the US, Canada, and Japan, and millions of cattle have been slaughtered to prevent the spread of the disease, which is transmitted through eating infected meat and bone meal. Someone joked that the result of this crisis was "the herd shot 'round the world." Others just ignore the risk, including cow brain lovers in places like Evansville, Indiana, where deep-fried cow brain sandwiches remain on the menu in some restaurants.[3]

The disease-causing agents in brains are called "prions," which are infectious proteins that cause microscopic holes in the brain. These proteins resist being broken down by the body's natural enzymes. Once infection happens, there is no treatment; the disease is uniformly fatal.[4]

Several other meat-borne diseases can affect your brain. Pork tapeworm has been around for thousands of years, and millions of people have it in their GI tract, mostly in the undeveloped world. Unless attached to feces, it cannot affect the brain. So in addition to being careful what you eat, be careful where you eat, and who prepares the food.

Trichinosis is another threat to your brain, as well as to your body. The 1982 Swedish biographical drama *Flight of the Eagle* (nominated for the Academy Award for Best Foreign Language Film in 1983) was based on Per Olof Sundman's novelization of the true story of S.A. Andrée's Arctic balloon expedition of 1897, an ill-fated effort to reach the North Pole in which all three expedition members perished. Andrée and companions were trying to be the first to reach the North Pole using a hydrogen balloon, but the three were never heard from again. Their bodies were discovered thirty-three years later.

A detailed analysis of the evidence, including their journals, concluded that the cause of their deaths was not starvation or even freezing to death, but the ingestion of Trichinella parasites from undercooked meat from polar bears they had shot. Evidently, by the time of their deaths, the adventurers had experienced not only the typical digestive trouble, general illness, and exhaustion that comes with trichinosis, but the parasites had passed the blood-brain barrier, thus infecting their brains, a rare result of ingesting undercooked infected meat.

So, if symptoms including fever, muscle soreness, pain and swelling around the eyes, thirst, profuse sweating, chills, weakness, fatigue or worse are not on your "bucket list" then skip the meat of animals that carry trichinosis. If, however, you wish to consume the meat of domestic or wild pigs, wild boar, bears, dogs, cats, rats, foxes, or wolves, you can reduce the risk of trichinosis by cooking potentially infected meat to an internal temperature of 159.8° F for at least one minute, which kills the parasite.[5]

Finally, if emulating a mad squirrel is also absent from your "bucket list," we suggest you pack your own gourmet snacks should you visit rural Kentucky during squirrel season. Emulating a happy squirrel is okay, but an objective observer might think you're nuts!

SHARPER BRAIN TIPS

- Avoid exposure to *Trichinella*. You don't really have to eat *anything* that might expose you.
- Be careful where and what you eat, and be especially aware of who prepared it and how.
- Cook your meat thoroughly, avoid unpasteurized milk, and take care when exposed to cat feces. *Toxoplasma gondii* can cause "brain worms." This is why pregnant women should not clean cat litter boxes. You should also prevent cats from using children's sandboxes as potties.
- Skip pork for another reason—*Taenia solium*, the pork tapeworm.
- Practice what your mother said: "Cleanliness is next to godliness."

20

This is Your Brain On . . . Any Questions?

A mind is a terrible thing to waste.
— *United Negro College Fund*

THE FIVE MOST COMMON MIND-WASTING SUBSTANCES IN the US are: alcohol, marijuana, cocaine, heroin, and methamphetamine. All five contribute to physical, emotional, and relational catastrophe on an individual level, while placing a tremendous financial burden upon families and society. If you are in the family or social network of someone who uses one or more of these substances, you know, better than most, the meaning of the word "havoc."

These substances affect the brain chemistry by altering the level of neurotransmitters, which send signals throughout the brain and body, controlling thoughts, behavior, and emotions. They especially affect the neurotransmitter dopamine, reducing feelings of pain and increasing feelings of pleasure or well-being, even euphoria, while creating a craving for more.

Alcohol is the number one drug problem in the United States.

Alcohol dulls the mind, reducing pain and creating an artificial feel-good effect. While no one knows why some people can drink alcohol and not become alcoholics, there are many who start drinking and end up in slavery to the craving that ensues. If one were to believe Hollywood or TV advertising, alcohol consumption enhances social relationships and the pursuit of happiness (even if it is both false and transitory). Alcohol-impaired driving contributes to more than 10,000 highway deaths annually. Alcohol-impaired living contributes to an untold number of relational issues, including divorce.[1] Physically, alcohol puts a strain on the liver and pancreas as these organs try to clear the toxin from the body. Permanent damage can occur. Serious harm can also come to the kidneys, heart, brain, and central nervous system. Alcohol irritates and can eventually cause cancer of the stomach, mouth, throat, larynx, and esophagus. Does this sound like a good thing?

Marijuana takes control of the brain when the chemical, tetrahydrocannabinol (THC), binds with targets on brain cells called cannabinoid receptors, replacing the good chemicals called endocannabinoids. These receptors play an important role in brain development and function to influence memory, thinking, sensory and time perception, as well as coordination. The "high" that results from smoking marijuana distorts thinking and problem-solving abilities and disrupts learning and memory. Research clearly shows that heavy use leads to a plethora of physical, mental, and relational problems. Among other consequences, a profound deficit in connections between learning and memory can occur, as well as obesity from the interruption of natural occurring appetite control mechanisms. This is what some states have legalized. Does it sound like a good thing?

Cocaine presents itself in disguise as the "caviar of street drugs," so named because so many celebrities fall prey to it. Cocaine is causing long-term life-threatening consequences and sudden death across our country. Extracted from the erythroxylum coca bush, chemical processes produce powdered cocaine (coke) which is snorted or injected, or crack, which can be smoked. Cocaine quickly travels to the brain where it blocks many neurotransmitters from being reabsorbed, allowing for a toxic soup of chemicals to build up to dangerous levels between the brain cells, causing euphoria. Along with the "high" there can also be anxiety, paranoia, and irritability. Do these sound like good things?

Heroin can be injected, inhaled, or smoked. In 2011, 4.2 million Americans aged 12 or older had used heroin at least once in their lives.[3] Heroin rapidly targets the receptors in the reward center of the brain as well as areas in the brain-stem that control automatic body functions like breathing and blood pressure. The initial rush that occurs also clouds mental functioning and is quickly followed by a period of drowsiness ("on the nod"). Overdoses can cause cessation of breathing and death. Heroin is highly addictive and long-term effects are numerous including: collapsed veins, heart infections, liver, or kidney disease. As with other drugs like cocaine, babies born to addicted mothers can be negatively affected in many ways. This is not a good thing.

Methamphetamine is a white powder, dissolved and taken by mouth, snorted, smoked, or injected. Meth changes the dopamine level in the brain by increasing the amount released and then preventing its reabsorption, which produces an intense euphoria or "rush." Since this affects the way the brain functions, it can negatively affect emotion, memory, thinking, and motor skills, and it can cause irregular heartbeat, high blood pressure, and hyperthermia. Paranoia and violent behavior can occur. Even after meth use is stopped, these effects can persist. These also are not good things.

But even people who know that it's not a good thing to expose their brains to any of these substances can become entangled by one of them, usually alcohol. Bruce, a pastor in New England, started his slide toward alcohol dependence with one beer a week, usually after all the services of his church were over on Sunday evening. Over time, one beer became two; two became a six-pack. About three years into his descent, Bruce grew concerned with calorie intake (he was developing a "beer belly"), so he switched to vodka, because it was cheaper and less discernable in public (so he had heard), while expecting that vodka would give him the relief he sought for half the calories of Bud Light. Fairly soon, he was mixing it with Fresca for lunch, assuming that nobody would notice. Gradually, like all addicts, his craving came to dictate his days as well as his nights. He became a master of deceit, and his wife became increasingly concerned.

Ultimately, Bruce had to learn the long, hard lesson that only a more intimate relationship with the Lord could fill the void he was trying to fill illicitly. And he had to re-embrace the Lord's calling to love God and the people around him with all his heart (i.e. more than he had come to love the bottle) in order to finally break free, while still fighting the craving day-by-day, as all addicts must. "I hated the taste of vodka," he admits in retrospect. "But I loved the way it made me feel. But now . . . now I know that feeling was just another form of anesthesia, and that life without the fog is far better."

SHARPER BRAIN TIPS

- If you are concerned that you may be addicted to a substance, do not hesitate to solicit help from an addiction professional.
- If someone you care about is abusing substances, focus on positive ideas and directions. It is highly unlikely that either nagging or shaming will motivate any substance abuser to recover, long-term.
- Enlist positive people who understand the issues to be part of your support team.
- Identify unique activities that can bring a natural high to replace the imposters—sports, hobbies, friendships, new projects, a healthy church experience. These can all provide a dopamine boost.
- Don't start. That first drink is your worst enemy.

21

Stick to Quiet Fish

"Eat that fish. It's brain food!" – *School Lunch Cook, 1966*

WHEN I (DAVE) WAS GROWING UP, FRIDAY WAS FISH DAY in the school hot lunch program in our little Vermont town. So, on Fridays in school, we got some sort of fish—fish sticks, fish cakes, cod, flounder, scrod, ocean perch, sea bass, or whatever the government source of surplus fish had to unload that month. Strange, we never got gefilte fish.

Some of the kids seemed content to eat what was served on Fridays, perhaps because their moms had told them the same thing that my mom told me—fish is brain food. Looking back now, I wonder that none of us asked for double-blind, placebo-controlled scientific evidence to prove that eating fish was any better for our brains than a PB&J sandwich on white bread (sometimes with marshmallow worked in), or burger and fries, with onion rings and a big Coke.

All jesting aside, I'm glad my mom and the school lunch cook made us eat our fish, because now there is a mountain of gold standard scientific evidence that eating fish can enhance brain health. What nobody knew at the time, however, was that some fish can retain heavy metals, such as mercury, which are toxic to the brain. In general, the higher up the food chain the fish, the more likely it is to be contaminated by mercury, since the metal accumulates over time.

Piscatorially speaking, feeding your brain well may involve *learning* to like fish, with wild caught oily cold water fish being superior because of their ability to deliver Omega-3 fatty acids, which the human body needs but cannot produce on its own. Omega-3s are important throughout life, helping to maintain brain function, and may have a significant role in protecting your brain from some effects of aging. Omega-3s can be obtained from a variety of plant sources, but the most common source is fish, including wild salmon, high mountain trout or other cold water trout, mackerel, herring, sardines, and anchovies.

I've shared this message in various ways with various folks, some of whom instantly reply, "But I don't like fish!" The only rational reply to that would be, "But do you like your mind and want to keep it?"

Then if all you can elicit is an adamant, "Yuk," you might suggest that if the person simply will not consume fish, but they do want some of the benefits, a variety of fish oils can be purchased locally or via the Internet—just to be sure that whatever they ingest is certified free of all toxins. In addition, they need to be aware that the scientific jury is still out regarding the efficacy of Omega-3 in supplement form.

Some doctors recommend eating a half-pound of fish every week,[1] this despite the relatively disturbing report issued by the US government which showed that fish in all of the nearly 300 streams sampled over a seven-year period contained mercury to some degree, although only about 25 percent had mercury levels exceeding what the EPA considers safe for people consuming average amounts of fish.

"Mercury consumed by eating fish can damage the nervous

system and cause learning disabilities in developing fetuses and young children," the report said. "The main source of mercury to most of the streams tested, according to the researchers, is emissions from coal-fired power plants. The mercury released from smokestacks here and abroad rains down into waterways, where natural processes convert it into methylmercury—a form that allows the toxin to wind its way up the food chain into fish."

Some fish and shellfish are contaminated with polychlorinated biphenyls or PCBs. PCBs are man-made pollutants that, although they are no longer manufactured in the US, have gotten into the environment. PCBs and other contaminants concentrate in the fat of fish just underneath the skin. Other contaminants include dioxins and pesticides. If you eat fish that you catch, you should check your local fish consumption advisory at the EPA web site: *www.epa.gov/waterscience/fish/states*.

Fish that tend to have higher levels of mercury include shark, swordfish, king mackerel, and tilefish.[2] Fish typically low in mercury include shrimp, canned light tuna, salmon, and catfish. You can prepare fish to reduce the levels of contaminants, for example, by removing the skin and fat before you cook the fish. You can then bake or broil the fish on a rack so that the fat containing the contaminants drips away from the fish.

Studies show that aging people in some countries who consume larger amounts of fish had reduced rates of dementia and reduced losses of mental functioning. And in other countries where people eat more fish, the rates of depression are lower.[3] So a good plan is to eat the right kind of fish, one or two meals per week, because the potential health benefits outweigh the potential negatives.

In case you're wondering, there is a way to tell if the fish on your plate contains heavy metal. Lean over, with one ear about an inch from the fish, and listen. If you hear loud noise pretending to be music, don't eat it. It's a heavy metal rock band fish.

SHARPER BRAIN TIPS

- If you have a choice between farmed or wild fish, wild may be safer, depending on its origin.
- If you can choose between imported versus domestic fish, domestic may be safer.
- If it is "farmed," look for the country of origin. US farm-raised fish are safer than foreign farm-raised fish due to varying international safety standards.
- If a package of fish claims to be "organic," inspect the label. For example, farm-raised "organic" Atlantic salmon are often imported from regions not certified by US standards.
- If you like "catfish," be sure that you are not buying imported fish of other species called "catfish" where they are raised. Stick to US farm-raised catfish.
- If you are concerned with conservation as well as safety, consume fish that are raised via "sustainable" fish farming.
- Make it your goal to become an informed fish consumer, and stick to "quiet" fish.

22

"Let's Go Surfing Now. . . ."

– The Beach Boys (1962)

BACK IN THE '60S, A FEW PEOPLE SURFED, THOUGH CATCHING a wave at Malibu was then, and still is, a not-for-everyone kind of sport. Today, if you ask someone if they've been "surfing" recently, most will say yes, but they'll have in mind the much tamer waves of the Internet.

Once upon a time, you had to go to the library to research anything. Just finding and copying a few good quotes from books or journals could take hours. Today, there is no doubt that the Internet has become *the* primary source of access to information on just about any topic imaginable, a lot of it free of charge.

Of all the books I (Dave) have helped create, the longest one took about 1 megabyte of disk space. Just now I sent it to myself as an e-mail attachment, to see how long two years' worth of wordsmithing takes to transfer from me to myself. Answer: 7.8 seconds.

Today's DVD disks will hold up to 4.7 gigabytes (GB) on one layer; a dual-layer DVD has a capacity of 8.7 GB of memory. Using 1 megabyte per book as an average, you could store nearly

5,000 books on a single one-layer DVD. That number used to be impressive, when one considered the lack of access to various kinds of books in some parts of the world. As I write, I have a 128-gigabyte USB flash drive plugged into one of the dozen or so USB ports built into or connected to my desktop computer. On that single flash drive, the length and width of which is about 3/4 inch by 2 1/4 inches, and the weight perhaps four ounces, you could store about 140,000 books. I have two 32-gigabyte SD cards that measure about 1 inch by 3/4 inch by 1/10th of an inch and weigh perhaps 1/20th of an ounce. Imagine 35,000 books stored on something not a whole lot larger than two thumbnails.

Impressive as it may seem to be able to carry the equivalent of a library in the watch pocket of your jeans, that size is still infinitesimal compared with the vast number of books that are *already* available for download via the Internet. All you need is an e-book reader compatible with the book service you're using, and you can order, download, store, and start to read a book of normal length in a minute or less, depending on your connection speed.

In really olden times, when we were kids, you could sign up for a "pen pal," and communicate with someone in a faraway place like France or Africa a few times a year by mail. Such a boring old world we (Dave, Jim, and Bobbie) lived in, growing up! Only books to read, board games to play, stories to tell around the campfire, letters and even essays of more than twenty-five words in length to write with no way to cut and paste, and mathematic calculations to perform without calculators. Today . . . all of these, including campfires (we're told) in some presentations by Park Rangers, are digitized. What a world! Let's make the most of it.

Today, you can communicate almost instantly with anyone who is "online" and whose e-mail address you have. You can "talk" back and forth using instant messaging programs. Or better yet, you can chat in real time with anyone anywhere in the world who has an account with Skype, which also allows the addition of real-time video so, with the right equipment, you can see the person you're talking with, and they can see you—or not, depending on your preferences and the status of your makeup. Recently, there were forty-eight million users logged on to Skype at the same time.

In less time than it took the Egyptians to build the Great Pyramid of Giza, the Internet, officially established in 1987, has become one of the greatest wonders this world has ever known. Today, you can buy almost anything online, whether you visit eBay, the world's largest auction "house," where a jet was sold for $4.7 million and a ghost in a jar fetched a nifty $50,922 (which the bidder never paid). You might visit Amazon.com, the world's largest online store, which started with books, but now carries just about anything anyone could want. You can buy nearly new books at Half.com for seventy-five cents plus shipping. You can buy prescription drugs online, without a prescription, from someplace overseas. You can buy clothes, athletic equipment, toys, pet supplies, office supplies, a college degree, a PhD, or even get yourself ordained via the Internet.

Perhaps even more importantly, the Internet has become the world's primary social networking and "chatting" place, thanks to millions of chat rooms on any subject imaginable, and instant communication with others using today's "smart" cell phones, which have amazing capabilities, including cameras offering still and video photography, GPS guidance, and as many "apps" (applications) as one could want, with more coming. Huge networks make it possible for *anyone* with Internet access, worldwide, to become aware of *anything* that is going on in the world, within seconds of the event in question having happened. For example, when US Airways Flight 1549 crash landed in the Hudson River, and all aboard survived, the *first* images broadcast from the site were captured not by news reporters dispatched to the scene, but by a cell phone camera of someone on a ferry rushing to the scene. Even before the passengers and crew were rescued, the photo was published worldwide using TwitPic, a division of Twitter.

In retrospect, I feel like all these years of writing, editing, and web surfing, since I got my first computer in the early 80s, have kept my mind as sharp as it can be as I head toward a different kind of "80s," myself. One thing is for sure; thanks to computers and the Internet, I can't remember being bored, nor can I imagine what some of my contemporaries from our college class of 1970 are longing for—retirement. It's a wonderful age in which to be alive, and the Internet is part of the reason.

Yes, there are dangers in surfing, from Malibu to the Internet. But some very good times can be had, whether mastering the perfect pipeline wave, or coming up with the all-time highest Pathword score of anyone you know. It's all relative, in the end. But our suggestion is that in the best interest of keeping your mind sharp, you become as computer savvy as you can become, that you acquire the best equipment you can afford, and then learn to use it wisely and well, including how to safely and productively surf the Net, which will keep your synapses firing instead of retiring.

SHARPER BRAIN TIPS

- Learn what you can about the Internet, realizing that you do not have to understand it to use it.

- Adopt the perspective that the Internet is neither good nor evil; rather, it is a magnificent product of our digital age that can be extremely useful or very destructive.

- View the Internet as a giant web of connections—including personal computers to mainframes, cell phones, tablets, music players, GPS units, soda machines, auto tracking devices, dog collars, whole libraries of various things . . . the list keeps growing.

- Learn how to search the Internet effectively and efficiently. Develop your own approach toward sifting through billions of choices in order to find what you need. If you're obsessive about being comprehensive, you could search forever to find everything about anything.

23

Participate by Proxy

Games lubricate the body and the mind.
– Benjamin Franklin[1]

YOU'VE HAD A ROUGH WEEK AND ALL YOU WANT TO DO ON the weekend is veg out in front of the TV with your favorite snacks and watch your favorite sports shows. If anyone asked you what your favorite sport is, you might just say, "yes," because sometimes it really doesn't matter as long as you can lose yourself in the game, any game.

Ladies, you may be thinking, *That sounds just like my husband!* But according to a study done by Scarborough Sports Marketing, women are increasingly becoming more passionate about professional sports. The lure for women is the same as for men: exciting games and the opportunity to participate by proxy. So the next time you're at the ballpark or stadium, check it out—much of the crowd consists of women. Watching and participating in sports is no longer just a "guy thing," which in some cases could be a marriage-saver.

Participating in sports is good for you. Do you like to walk? How about beefing it up and starting to train for a half or full marathon? Running isn't a requirement—many people choose to walk the course.

Walking improves your ability to make decisions, solve problems, and to focus. It's also a great stress buster and you'll sleep better at night.

Aerobic activities release hormones, such as adrenaline and endorphins. These are good for your nervous system, boosting your mood, relieving pain, and creating a sense of well-being. Also, if you train with a friend, you're more likely to keep going, and the social connection is also good for your mental functioning.[2]

Let's say you're actively engaged in some kind of physical activity or sport, but still enjoy following your favorite team(s) on TV. Maybe it's the day of the big game and you invite some friends over to watch. You enjoy discussing the play-by-play, talking the language of the game, and, if it's football, being an armchair quarterback.

According to research conducted by the University of Chicago, you can improve brain functioning *both by participating in and by watching sports.* "Being an athlete or merely a fan improves language skills when it comes to discussing their sport because parts of the brain usually involved in playing sports are instead used to understand sport language.[3]

"For the study, researchers asked twelve professional and intercollegiate hockey players, eight fans and nine individuals who had never watched a game to listen to sentences about hockey players, such as shooting, making saves and being engaged in the game. They also listened to sentences about everyday activities, such as ringing doorbells and pushing brooms across the floor. While the subjects listened to the sentences, their brains were scanned using MRI, which allows one to infer the areas of the brain most active during language listening."

After hearing the sentences, the subjects were given tests that would gauge their understanding of those sentences. Most subjects understood the language about everyday activities, and it's reasonable that hockey players and fans understood hockey-related language better than the novices.[4]

The results showed "that a region of the brain usually associated with planning and controlling actions is activated when players and fans listen to conversations about their sport. The brain boost helps athletes' and fans' understanding of information about their sport and the language connected with it.

Playing sports, or even just watching, builds a stronger understanding of language. Brain areas usually used to act become highly involved in language understanding. There is a change in the neural networks that support comprehension in incorporating areas active in performing sports skills."[5]

Evidently, according to the research, it's okay to be hooked on watching your favorite sports, in moderation of course. Those small pleasures can translate into good health for your brain. So, grab a healthy snack, curl up on the couch, and watch that game (for now, let's imagine you're watching football):

- Engage yourself with the strategies and execution of various calls by the coaches and key players on offense and defense.
- Try to understand clock management, if it applies.
- Learn as many of the rules as your brain will tolerate.
- Turn the sound off from time to time, and see how many of the signals given by the officials you can understand without hearing what is said.
- Play the game in your mind as it progresses. Try to predict plays before they happen. This will take a thorough knowledge of both teams.
- Get inside the minds of the quarterback and his favorite receiver. At the same time, like playing yourself

in chess, plot the defensive strategy of the other team, and what each player's assignment might be.

While your favorite team may not win every game, it can still be fun and it can be healthy for the functioning of your brain.

SHARPER BRAIN TIPS

- Try watching the next "big game" with the sound off and some headphones on, with the music of Chopin playing as the game progresses, and your hands knitting (if you know how) or doing something else like typing or texting a message on your phone, even if you're just going to send it to yourself.
- Turn off the sound of the game you're watching, and take the roles of the play-by-play announcer or a cohort commentator whose job is to add "color" and to explain what's happening, including any calls that have been made by officials.
- Include a slower moving sport like golf, which is entertaining to watch and can even be brain-stretching if you mentally strategize and swing with each player, and deal with possible penalty strokes, for example.
- If you like baseball, keep score the old way, using a scoring book, and not relying on replays. You'll be amazed how that engages your mind with the game.
- Consider participating in a "fantasy" version of your favorite sport. This will not only STP your brain if you choose stock car racing, it will stimulate your mind and hone your computer skills regardless what sport you choose.
- Get your head into whatever game you're "playing by proxy"—from auto racing to Zui Quan—and see how much more you enjoy it.

24

Fertilize Your Mind

A strong link was found between physical activity and brain health . . . older people who exercise are less likely to experience cognitive decline. — *NIH Panel*[1]

Research shows that we are not total victims of our genes and that lifestyle, especially physical exercise, will help equip our brains for the journey before us. We have heard again and again that exercise breathes new life into almost every organ system in our body. Now we can add the brain to the list.

The connection between cardiovascular exercise and brain function has been studied by many teams who have concluded that moderate exercise triggers a release of neurotropins in the memory area (hippocampus) of the brain. Neurotropins promote growth and repair of neural tissue. Neurotropins have been studied in animals and are clearly shown to counteract the ravages of diseases affecting memory. Studies are underway to determine if physical exercise could delay symptoms in people who are at genetic risk for Alzheimer's disease.[2]

One of our physician friends wrote, in relation to his many aging patients who are worried about diminished mental acuity, "It turns out that physical exercise does more to prevent brain shrinkage in the hippocampus area than mental exercises. I believe totally in the 'use it or lose it theory,' but first keep it oxygenated with good circulation, then keep on playing bridge or chess or reading. Many studies back this up."

You may be thinking, *I am over fifty and don't exercise much. Isn't it too late to start?* Researchers assure us that it is never too late to begin to take advantage of all the benefits exercise has to offer. Not only will you delay mental decline, you will also likely notice an improvement in mood and more control over your response to stress.

A visit to a physician who is up to date on these findings is a good first step and he/she will guide you on your way to a good exercise regimen. You may be relieved to know that research has proven that, when it comes to exercise and the brain, harder is not necessarily better.

The most positive brain results are achieved through moderate exercise. In fact, animal studies have found that over-exercising is not good for the brain. The theory is that if too much of the body's stress hormones are produced, it retards the brain's ability to make new brain cells. For most people, doctors will usually recommend thirty- to forty-five-minute sessions of moderate exercise four or five days a week at 60 percent of your maximum pulse rate, unless of course you happen to be an elite athlete, in which case the target pulse rate will be higher.[3]

"Exercise optimizes the brain and the person for learning; it creates the right environment for all of our 100 billion nerve cells up there," says Dr. John Ratey, a professor of psychiatry at the Harvard Medical School and the author of *Spark*, a book that examines how our brains change when we exercise. "I call it 'miracle grow' for the brain or brain fertilizer, which helps the brain cells stay alive, live longer and it helps the learning process," Ratey said.[4]

This is true for kids as well as adults. We (Bobbie and Jim) had a great opportunity to observe this up close when we had the unexpected pleasure of being offered a temporary hospital assignment very close to our son and granddaughter's hometown. Spending three months immersed in our granddaughter Kendal's world brought new insights and immeasurable joy to every day!

We noticed right away as we picked her up from school that every fiber in her eight-year-old body was yearning to run and play, so we got to be kids again as we climbed monkey bars and played soccer and hide-and-seek! We did decline the offer to join her doing cartwheels and rolling down hills! After this kind of exercise, Kendal was ready to settle into her favorite place to do homework while Bobbie started dinner.

We noticed how quickly she breezed through the math and reading, happily perched, of all places, on top of the kitchen counter! From her lofty seat she could stretch or climb up and down a few times when a math problem needed some extra thought and we could cheer her on as she finished each page. It took the "work" out of making sure all the homework got done. And then she could even teach us some of her newly learned science facts.

We have taken this lesson from Kendal to heart and try to intersperse as much physical exercise into our day as possible by taking even short breaks from the intensity of our work and trying whenever possible to make our brain-friendly exercise sessions fun. In fact, let's take a spin around the block right now!

So, if you want to do just one thing to improve your brain's health . . . just move! It doesn't have to be climbing one of Colorado's "fourteener" mountains, or trying to do five miles on a treadmill when you haven't walked a full mile at one time in awhile. Every movement counts. You can even "work out" while sitting at your desk in your cubicle at work. There are books that will tell you how. And your work will improve as a result, which is what you should tell anyone who asks what's going on.

SHARPER BRAIN TIPS

- Ask your personal physician if you are healthy enough to engage in exercise that is moderate or greater in intensity.
- To measure your daily activity, obtain a good pedometer. You may be surprised to find how many steps you take just in the process of working day-by-day. One medical assistant we know said she logged over 17,000 steps in a single day! Many people average between 3,000 to 5,000 steps per day during their work hours.
- If you want to augment your starting number, thirty minutes of relatively brisk walking will add about 3,000 steps (about 1.5 miles).
- A round number that has become a benchmark for active adults is 10,000 steps per day (though the usefulness of this number is under scrutiny). A brisk pace will log 10,000 steps in about 90 minutes. If you do set "active" as a goal and you're starting from "sedentary," it's probably best to try to reach 10,000 steps per day incrementally.
- For whole-person exercise, take a walk with a friend, during which you might share a nutritious picnic lunch, while discussing one of the most recent books you've both read. If you focus on a book with spiritual significance and perhaps even add in a little prayer as you go, you'll get some good exercise, while experiencing stress reduction and a better connection with God. It's hard to beat that combination!

25

Eat the Rainbow

Americans get more of their antioxidants from coffee than any other dietary source.   — Joe Vinson, PhD[1]

FEEDING YOUR BRAIN WELL BEGINS IN CHILDHOOD AND CONtinues throughout life. Those fortunate to have a parent who insisted on the consumption of healthy foods usually develop life-long habits that enhance health and thwart disease. Those who are not so fortunate may develop childhood eating habits that are quite difficult to change.

So, if you're a parent of growing children, make it your mission to feed them as well as possible, and thus "program" their preferences for life. But even if you're middle-aged or older, and you've been living on fast food and junk food and processed food with all the trans fats, sugars, salts, additives, and preservatives that have helped them sell since about 1950, it's never too late to give your body a chance to repair itself, cell by cell—and thankfully, studies are showing that such repair can even occur in the brain.

Consuming a wide variety of whole foods—fruits, vegetables, grains, nuts and berries—regularly is the most brain-friendly approach. A summary of research published in the August 2009 issue of the *Journal of Alzheimer's Disease* states: "Researchers have investigated the relationship between fruit and vegetable intake, plasma antioxidant micronutrient status and cognitive performance in healthy subjects aged 45 to 102 years. The study results . . . indicate higher cognitive performance in individuals with high daily intake of fruits and vegetables. Subjects with a high daily intake (about 400g) of fruits and vegetables had higher antioxidant levels, lower indicators of free radical-induced damage against lipids, as well as better cognitive performance compared to healthy subjects of any age consuming low amounts (<100g/day) of fruits and vegetables. Modification of nutritional habits aimed at increasing intake of fruits and vegetables, therefore, should be encouraged to lower the prevalence of cognitive impairment."[2]

Recently, science has been uncovering evidence that the micronutrients in whole foods help fight "oxidative stress," increasingly being blamed for contributing to degenerative diseases including those of the heart and brain. Today, entire antioxidant supplement empires sell wonder products from açaí berries to superchocolate. But did you know that their claims are built on a theory that is only about a half-century old?

The free radical theory of aging was proposed by Denham Harman in the 1950s, ". . . when prevailing scientific opinion held that free radicals were too unstable to exist in biological systems, and before anybody had invoked free radicals as a cause of degenerative diseases."[3] Here's just another example of how yesterday's unreasonable theory becomes tomorrow's maxim. In fact, one online document describing "Power Foods: Doctors' Top Choices for Antioxidant Rich Foods," begins with this sentence: "It's common knowledge that antioxidants protect us from dangerous substances called free radicals that can lead to many chronic diseases. Science touts antioxidants and their role in everything from preventing cancer and heart disease to boosting the immune system and slowing the aging process."[4] Claims like this plant an "antioxidants prevent disease" seed in the minds of otherwise uninformed consumers, many of whom prefer consuming capsules versus obtaining their essential nutrients from whole food. This, despite statements from various authorities that consuming antioxidants in the form of supplements has little measurable positive effect, and can be harmful.[5]

Keeping these things in mind, here's some food for thought— a list of important antioxidants and the foods that can best provide them:

- **Beta-carotene:** apricots, cantaloupe, carrots, mangos, pumpkin, sweet potatoes, and some green leafy vegetables including collard greens, kale, and spinach. (These three leafy vegetables also contain Lutein, essential to eye health.)
- **Lycopene:** apricots, blood oranges, guava, papaya, pink grapefruit, tomatoes, watermelon.
- **Vitamin A:** carrots, egg yolks, liver, milk, mozzarella cheese.
- **Vitamin C:** fruits and vegetables, as well as cereals, beef, poultry, and fish.
- **Vitamin E:** almonds, broccoli, mangos.

In general, what's good for your heart is good for your brain, because both depend on good blood flow. That's one reason why The Alzheimer's Association and the American Heart Association, along with its American Stroke Association division, launched a public awareness program to help African-Americans manage their heart and brain health (African-Americans are at greater risk than Caucasians for developing diabetes, Alzheimer's, vascular dementia, and stroke). The program is called "What's good for your heart is good for your head."[6]

Quoting just a bit from this program: "Some of the strongest evidence about maintaining your brain links brain health to heart health. Even though you can't feel your brain working, it's one of the most active organs in your body. Your heart pumps about 20 percent of your blood to your brain, where billions of cells use about 20 percent of the blood's oxygen and fuel."

SHARPER BRAIN TIPS

Many people think they eat enough fruits and vegetables; very few actually do. Even vegans have their favorite foods. In order to get the broad spectrum of whole food nutrients your brain needs, you have to "eat the rainbow." Here's a starter list:

<u>RED</u>
Beets
Cherries
Cranberries
Pomegranate
Radish
Raspberries
Red Apple
Red bell pepper
Strawberries
Tomatoes

<u>ORANGE</u>
Apricot
Butternut squash
Cantaloupe
Carrots
Kumquats
Mango
Nectarine
Orange
Peach
Sweet Potatoes
Tangerine

<u>YELLOW</u>
Corn
Lemon
Passion fruit
Pears
Pineapple
Plantains
Quince
Yellow squash

<u>GREEN</u>
Artichokes
Asparagus
Avocados
Bok Choy
Broccoli
Celery
Cucumbers
Edamame
Green beans
Green cabbage
Green grapes
Green pears
Green peppers
Honeydew melons
Kale
Kiwi
Leafy greens
Peas
Spinach
Sprouts
Zucchini

<u>BLUE (including PURPLE)</u>
Blueberries
Acai
Boysenberries
Eggplant
Fig
Purple grapes
Purple plums
Shallots
Turnip

Choose one fruit or vegetable from each list to brighten your meals today. Better—limit yourself to those you've never had before.

26

Rot Not Thy Brain

Because I only have got one brain to rot I'm gonna spend my life watching television a lot.
                           – From "Couch Potato" by Weird Al Yankovic

You've heard the term "couch potato," and maybe you are one, but do you know the phrase's origin? According to Answers.com, "Very few words have a birthday so precisely known as *couch potato*. It was on July 15, 1976, we are told, that *couch potato* came into being, uttered by Tom Iacino of Pasadena, California, during a telephone conversation. He was a member of a Southern California group humorously opposing the fads of exercise and healthy diet in favor of vegetating before the TV and eating junk food (1973). Because their lives centered on television—the boob tube (1966)—they called themselves *boob tubers*. Iacino apparently took the brilliant next step and substituted *potato* as a synonym for *tuber*. Thinking of where that potato sits to watch the tube, he came up with couch potato."

This history is important because, as the explanation adds, ". . . when the new phrase reached the ears of Robert Armstrong, another member of the boob tubers, he drew a cartoon of a potato on a couch, formed a club called the Couch Potatoes, registered the trademark and began merchandising Couch Potato paraphernalia, from T-shirts to dolls. He published a newsletter called *The Tuber's Voice: The Couch Potato Newsletter* and a book, *Dr. Spudd's Etiquette for the Couch Potato*.[1]

Quite often, couch potatoes are stereotyped as overweight, slovenly men sitting around in their underwear watching a variety of events on TV, downing potato chips and other trans-fat-laden snack foods with the help of a steady supply of beer.

The term entered the Oxford English Dictionary in 1993 and is so well known in the UK that a plan of the Prime Minister's Strategy Unit tied attempts "to combat the couch potato culture" to "[improving the UK's] international sporting performance."[2]

Athletic performance aside, perhaps more important to the general population is the impact of the couch potato culture on brain performance.

In her article "Is Your Brain a Couch Potato?" San Francisco Internist and columnist "Doc Gurley" writes, "our brain is not static. As we age, the rule of 'use it or lose it' becomes all important to your brain—but improvements have been documented at every age, and even after injury. Brains crave novel, challenging 'out of your comfort zone' activities to thrive."[3]

This premise has spawned a whole new industry of "brain fitness products," which seek to provide whole brain stimulation. "They include a variety of exercises targeting different types of cognitive abilities including memory, attention, language skills, visual skills and reasoning.

They represent an evolution of the classic paper-based options such as crosswords puzzles, word search and Sudoku. They may be more effective than their paper-based cousins for several reasons: (a) they present more novelty, (b) they are more varied, (c) they are usually more challenging and (d) they can be tailored to the user's performance."[4]

But how do you know which brain fitness products work? Answering that question has spawned new books. In *The SharpBrains Guide to Brain Fitness*, authors Alvaro Fernandez and Dr. Elkhonon Goldberg state, "Brain fitness is our brain's ability to readily create additional connections between neurons, and even to promote new neurons in certain parts of the brain. Research in neuropsychology and neuroscience shows that vigorous mental activity can lead to good brain fitness, which in turn, translates into a sharper memory, faster processing of information, better attention, and other improved cognitive skills. If the brain is flexible and molded through experience, the question is, 'What tools can help provide the right kind of experience to help refine our brains, from a structural and functional point of view?'"[5]

The authors go on to list their top twenty-one picks of brain training software, organized by purpose, including eight brain maintenance products, eight targeted brain workout products, and five stress management products, with *only two of the five stress management products having "medium-high" scores for "clinical validation."*

In other words, while the scientific jury is still out on most such products, a few have been validated already. It seems reasonable to expect that future studies will show that some similar products also promote brain health.

The main thing to keep in mind is that you can choose to challenge your mind versus veg'ing out, and if you do so, day by day, year after year, your brain won't "rot," as Al Yankovic says, but it will remain sharp and fit until you don't need it anymore.

SHARPER BRAIN TIPS

- Brain Age: This handheld device provides good fun at low cost. It is a worthy alternative to videogames, and an advancement on crossword puzzles or Sudoku.

- BrainWare Safari: This program is designed to train forty-one cognitive skills among kids aged 6-12 in a multimedia gaming format.

- FitBrains.com: A subscription gives access to tools for continued motivation and engagement, such as competitions, collaborative games, and frequent feedback.

- Happy-Neuron.com: Scientific Brain Training offers on-line games, plus several CD-Rom based games. The CD includes thirty-five games, five for the Nintendo Wii.

- Lumosity.com: Lumos Labs' web site presents an engaging online experience. It may provide a good value-per-dollar for anyone with high-speed Internet access and a general "mental sharpening" goal.

- MindFit: This is the only software with an embedded stand-alone and comprehensive assessment of fourteen different cognitive skills, used to tailor the program to the user's needs.

- (m)Power Brain Fitness: This product is specially designed for retirement communities and people not familiar with computers. It includes a touch-screen system and the content is fun.

- Try "brain training" to address your brain's craving for novel things.

27

You Can Go Home Again

Tell me the story often, for I forget so soon; the early dew of morning has passed away at noon.[1]
— *Hymn lyrics by A. Katherine Hankey*

PERHAPS YOU'VE WONDERED WHY SO MANY OLDER FOLKS attend church so regularly. Is it a social issue—to be with other people and thus counter their feelings of loneliness or isolation? Is it a salvation issue—a way to try to earn divine credits with the One they're likely to meet sooner than later? A psychological issue—to receive encouragement, hope, and inner peace? A way to insure a church burial when the time comes? A way to feel better about themselves, at least for awhile? Or is it to strengthen their faith as well as their minds? Faith, yes, most likely, but minds? Can church attendance strengthen the mind?

Research indicates that it can, slowing cognitive decline in the healthy and further decline in those who already have Alzheimer's disease. "Results showed that religious attendance, not religious identity, was associated with a reduction in the odds of cognitive dysfunction over time. Compared with those who attended religious services less than once per week, those who attended services once per week or more exhibited a 36% reduction in the odds of cognitive dysfunction over 3 years."[2]

The same article added, "Results showed that higher levels of religiosity and religious practice were associated with slower rates of cognitive decline in Alzheimer's patients. The researchers concluded that spirituality and religious practices may delay the progression of Alzheimer's disease."[3]

Although no one knows for sure the mechanism that produces these positive results, they are consistent with other data about the longevity benefits of church attendance and the active pursuit of personal faith by other methods. Our own theory is that the whole experience of church attendance—including the social, psychological, and spiritual connections that occur during worship—may strengthen the biological connections known as synapses in the brain.

Don is in his sixties. When he attends a church similar to that of his youth, his connections to his lifelong faith are renewed, along with his sense of hope and even optimism that comes when one rests in the sovereignty of God during difficult times. "My dad was a Baptist minister," Don said, "so we were in church whenever the doors were open. Week after week, year after year, like the changing seasons, we heard the Scriptures read from the 'Authorized Version,' and we sang our way through the Baptist hymnal.

Since neither of these has changed much in a half-century, when I attend church now, I can still sing most of those hymns, from memory, and recite a lot of the Scripture, too. Even some of the sermons seem familiar, though deliveries and personalities vary from preacher to preacher. In any case, at the end of many Sunday morning services, I feel like I've been 'home again,' in some way reconnected with what is not just familiar, but really real. Yes, sometimes I am reminded of my shortcomings, but that makes the grace of God even more special. I believe all these things clear my mind and help me focus better on what is really important in the week to come."

Other areas of investigation may show similar results from less public religious activities, including devotional reading or participation in small study groups. While these would be harder to quantify scientifically than discovering how often a person attends public services, there is enough evidence to show that reading can significantly reduce stress, so spiritual activities involving reading seem logical candidates for improving or sustaining one's brain health.

When you add in group discussion of what one has found during one's devotional reading over the past week, the social dimension kicks in again, in addition to the stimulation of your mind through sharing your thoughts and listening to others express theirs. This is one modern way to accomplish what the apostle Paul instructed his own disciple, Timothy, to do; specifically, to stir up the gift of God that was in him (most likely a reference to his faith, which had been passed on to him by his mother and grandmother), "For God hath not given us the spirit of fear; but of power, and of love, and of a sound mind" (2 Tim. 1:7, KJV).

In small groups, sometimes called "house churches," all around the world, believers are stirring up each other's faith, thus increasing the strength of their beliefs, their love for one another, and the serious-mindedness that comes from viewing things from an eternal versus a temporal perspective.

So, however you can accomplish it, it surely makes sense to hear some part of "the old, old story" on a regular basis. And it also seems reasonable to do all we can to help our aging friends or relatives participate with us as often as possible. After all, the spiritual needs of your mother or grandmother have not diminished with aging, and their cognitive abilities may benefit from attending "church" with you, more than you can imagine.

SHARPER BRAIN TIPS

- Memorize Scripture: Start with John 3:16.
- Memorize words of hymns: This occurs through repetition—the lyrics go to the mind; the music carries them to the heart.
- Participate in topical studies and discussion groups: These can help expand your perspective, stimulate your thinking, deepen your knowledge, and even challenge your values and opinions.
- Remember: "Remember" occurs 231 times in the NIV translation of the Bible. Perhaps the best known use of this concept came from Jesus, himself, at the Last Supper, when he said, "Do these things in remembrance of me."
- Renew your mind, week by week, through worship.

28

Stop and Smell the Memories

How sense-luscious the world is.   – *Diane Ackerman*[1]

WHEN YOU THINK OF NOSES, *WHO* COMES TO MIND? Cyrano de Bergerac, De Gaulle, or Pinocchio, perhaps. But how about Mehmet Ozyurek of Turkey, whose nose is the longest in the world, at 4.5 inches? When you think of noses, *what* comes to mind? Nose hair, nose warts, sneezes, snorts, runny noses, sniffling noses, blowing noses, itchy noses, nose picking, nose wrinkling, or laying a finger aside one's nose, as with Santa in the famous poem, or with others, worldwide, who use this gesture to show that they share with you some secret that must remain that way.

Or maybe you think of nose jokes like, "Your nose is so big, the only date you can get is with an anteater." Or, "I've got it all backward today. My nose is running and my feet smell."

Whoever or whatever comes to mind, your nose is no joke, and keeping it "clean" is important to the health of your body, including your brain. We breathe about 23,000 times a day, often with our mouth closed. The healthier your nose, the better your oxygenation. Beyond that, a healthy nose is crucial to your sensory enjoyment of food, flowers, and perfume, among many other things.

As Diane Ackerman wrote, "Nothing is more memorable than a smell. One scent can be unexpected, momentary and fleeting, yet conjure up a childhood summer beside a lake in the mountains; another, a moonlit beach; a third, a family dinner of pot roast and sweet potatoes during a myrtle-mad August in a Midwestern town. Smells detonate softly in our memory like poignant land mines hidden under the weedy mass of years. Hit a tripwire of smell and memories explode all at once. A complex vision leaps out of the undergrowth."[2]

It is fairly common for people to experience a loss of smell in life, temporarily. This could be from a sinus problem, a cold, or allergies. If you've ever noticed a diminished sense of taste, you were really experiencing a loss of smell. When you eat and drink, most of what you sense is due to aroma rather than taste. You can differentiate four basic tastes (sweet, salty, sour, and bitter) but you can smell a large number of different odors. When you eat and swallow food, odors in your mouth are released to travel to your nose through a back passageway, enhancing your sense of taste.

Anosmia is the loss of the sense of smell. While it has many causes, exposure to toxic chemicals, allergies, and infections can bring it on. The olfactory bulb lies near the base of your brain at the top of your nose, between your eyes. The olfactory bulb can be damaged, or the olfactory nerve that carries the messages to your brain can be damaged. The damage can lead to a loss of smell.

Anosmia can be temporary or permanent. Medical researchers have been studying possible links between chemicals that gain access to the olfactory system, such as by inhalation of vapors or dusts, and the loss of smell. The loss of the sense of smell can be life-threatening because if you lose your sense of smell you will not be able to detect dangerous chemicals—during a gas leak, for example.

The loss of your sense of smell could signal problems with your brain, including some neurodegenerative diseases.[3] "Researchers at the University of Pennsylvania School of Medicine have linked smell loss in mice with excessive levels of a key protein associated with Alzheimer's and Parkinson's disease. Smell loss is well documented as one of the early and first clinical signs of such diseases. If smell function declines as the levels of this protein increase in brain regions associated with smelling, the research could validate the use of smell tests for diagnosing Alzheimer's disease.

Although everyone tends to slowly lose their sense of smell as they age, scratch and sniff tests have been developed for doctors to use to determine if someone is losing their sense of smell earlier than normal.[4]

There is a zone on your face called the "danger triangle."[5] It extends from the two corners of your mouth up to the top of your nose and includes your nose. Infections that develop in this area can, though rarely, flow directly to your brain via the blood supply and the cavernous sinus. Even infections of your upper front teeth are included in this danger triangle.

To protect yourself from infections in your nose, make sure that any water that enters your nose is safe, such as sterile saline water designed and sold for that purpose.

Second, protect against infections in the danger triangle on your face. See a doctor early on if you have questions about possible infected sites. Meanwhile, keep your nose clean, but let's not keep the importance of nose health a secret!

And remember, as your mother always said, you can pick your friends and you can pick your nose, but you can't pick your friend's nose.

SHARPER BRAIN TIPS

- For a fun project, keep track of your ability to smell as you get older.
  - Create a notebook to use for this multi-year self-study.
  - Select foods that have distinct smells, such as canned corn, sliced apples, peaches, and peeled bananas. Avoid foods with spicy type sensations, such as onion and clove, as these can trick you into thinking you smell them when it is not their smell that you are detecting.
  - Outdoor items such as roses and cut grass have a strong and distinctive odor. Include these and other "wild things" in your olfactory experiment. Include some vegetables from the garden if you have one.
  - In one column, list the categories of the origins of the scents you will be tracking. Once a year, record your observations. Note how strongly each item smells to you: for example—strong smelling, easy to smell, difficult to smell, can't smell. Over time, if you notice a trend of loss in smell function, talk to your doctor about it.
- Don't let your "danger triangle" become a Bermuda triangle.

29

Can You Say, "Talafa Lava"?

A different language is a different vision of life.
    – Federico Fellini, Italian film director

As children, many of us enjoyed watching a spy movie where the hero or heroine easily passes through enemy checkpoints by speaking a foreign language fluently. You may even have fantasized about being a multilingual world traveler. Now you think that time has slipped away from you and, with it, so has your fantasy. But not so fast! It turns out that learning another language might not only fulfill your childhood dream, it may also provide your brain with a workout regimen that will help keep it sharp into the endgame of life. Learning a language exercises a unique part of the brain, and it is different for reading and for conversation. Like cross-training, it exercises a different set of "brain muscles."

Perhaps as a child you heard someone say that they tried to learn a new language when they were in school, but it was just too hard. So you thought, *If it was too hard for mom and dad when they were my age, it's probably also too hard for me.* What may have been true for them is not necessarily true for you. One of the largest and most reliable longitudinal health studies, conducted by the Boston University School of Medicine, was launched in 1948 and studied 5,209 healthy adults living in Framingham, Massachusetts. The original study, called "The Framingham Study," gave birth to a study of the children of those in the original study.

Since 1971, this second study, which is called "The Framingham Offspring Study," has shown, among other things, that the "Framingham offspring perform approximately 1 standard deviation better than their parents on most memory tests administered at comparable ages, despite (on average) sharing the same genes."[1]

In separate studies, it has been observed that the average IQ in the US increases by about 3 points every decade.[2] The good news is that your parents' boundaries are not yours. You are likely to live longer[3] and, based on choices you can make, you can do it with a cognitively younger brain.

While it is true that young brains easily make new connections, which facilitates learning, a Johns Hopkins University team recently published a study demonstrating that new adult-born neurons have a youthful level of plasticity, but only for a limited time window. They observed that this "represent[s] not merely a replacement mechanism for lost neurons but instead an ongoing developmental process that continuously rejuvenates the mature nervous system by offering expanded capacity of plasticity in response to experience throughout life."[4]

Another barrier to learning a new language is that, as you have aged, you have unconsciously developed acute listening "filters" to help your brain focus in on those parts of verbal expressions that carry most of the meaning. These filters include factors like inflection, emphasis on syllables, intensity, pauses, tone of voice, and so forth.

The trick about learning a new language is accepting that the English "filters" that you have been training for decades may not serve you well when learning a new language, because the information is carried differently. For example, in English you're used to hearing emphases placed on certain syllables, or a certain type of inflection or tone when someone has finished a particular sentence. Other languages you want to learn may use entirely different inflections or tones. So, be patient with yourself. It will take time to un-train your English filters and train your subconscious for new language filters.

Bobbie recalls, "Our language filters, as well as those of our patients, were certainly in place on our first day of clinic in American Samoa as we strove to cross the wide language barrier. Samoans are remarkable, gentle, and resilient people who were warm and receiving, but many spoke little, if any, English. We, on the other hand, spoke no Samoan other than *talafa lava* (hello) and *tofa soifua* (goodbye)!

"That first day we quickly learned that if we were to make any progress toward helping our patients, we most definitely needed an interpreter to discern where the 'pain in the belly' was coming from. By the end of the week we had made many new friends and learned some pronunciations and meanings in this beautiful language.

"The children taught us some Samoan songs and we saw firsthand how much it means to a person of another culture when a visitor attempts to speak their native language. On our last day we participated in a Samoan church service where all attendees from youngest baby to eldest Auntie were dressed in white and we were blessed by hearing our familiar hymns and choruses sung in Samoan by the villagers."

SHARPER BRAIN TIPS

- If you speak English, don't start with Mandarin Chinese, unless you'll be visiting China soon and want a head start.
- Start with Spanish or French, with a good teacher, and you'll feel "les cellules du cerveau" multiply!
- Combine new language learning with other strategies for brain health. For example, social interaction is good for brain health. If you learn your language by going to evening school, perhaps at the local high school, you will be interacting with others who are also struggling to "unlearn" their English filters, just like you. You and your fellow struggling students may form a new social network.
- Celebrate every new level reached as your journey toward polyglotism continues.
- Make your new motto, "No strain, no brain!"
- Refuse to give up if the learning gets rough. After all, if young children can learn that language, so can you!
- When you can say *talafa lava* (hello) and *tofa soifua* (goodbye), you'll be as ready as we were to visit American Samoa.

30

"Water, Water Everywhere ... nor any drop to drink"[1]

Once we can secure access to clean water and adequate sanitation facilities for all people, irrespective of the difference in their living conditions, a huge battle against all kinds of diseases will be won. – Dr. Lee Jong-wook, Director-General World Health Organization[2]

OKAY. YOU'RE STANDING ON THAT SCALE AGAIN, CONVINCED that it must be off by at least ten pounds of ugly fat. Or maybe it's water. After all, 60–70 percent of your total weight is water. About 90 percent of your blood is water. About 75 percent of your brain is water.

Water is essential for your life. But too much water (water intoxication), as well as too little water (dehydration) can affect your brain and in severe cases even lead to death. That is why it is crucial to drink sufficient amounts of clean water every day and to avoid contaminated water as much as possible.

Children, especially, need clean water, since they are often more vulnerable than adults to problems with drinking water because their bodies and brains are developing. This need has led to testing tap water in schools and daycare centers.[3]

Problems with unclean water have occurred across the country for a variety of reasons: corroded plumbing of large school buildings, poor water quality of country schools that obtain water from private wells, and under-maintained conditions of large and small daycare centers. These conditions can result in elevated levels of lead and copper.

Concerned parents should first discuss this with the educational facility's persons in charge. Some water testing may have already been done. Certified laboratories can be contacted to provide water testing, if needed. In all cases, there should be recent information about the safety of the tap water. Additional concerns can always be directed to the state's environmental health officers or the US Environmental Protection Agency (EPA). EPA's Safe Drinking Water Hotline is 1-800-426-4791.

Do you take your tap water for granted? That is, do you expect that every time you turn on the kitchen faucet, clean, drinkable water will come flowing out? Do you also take water for granted when you bathe and shower—when you immerse yourself beneath the safe, warm water and wash your face? This is true for most Americans, even though a recent report found that bathroom shower heads are often a breeding ground for bacteria.[4]

Worldwide, many people would be happy just to have a shower head to sanitize; instead, they don't even have access to safe, clean water if they have running water at all. In 2004, the World Health Organization reported that over one million people die every year from water-related diseases, most of them children under five years of age in countries where safe water and sanitation are lacking. So if you're traveling abroad, you need to check with travel experts about the safety of the tap water at your destination, and if necessary, take along appropriate treatment options or filtration systems to protect your health, in general, and your brain in particular.[5] Of course the safest choice is to not drink any of the local water.

We (Bobbie and Jim) can attest to this when, on a recent medical trip to American Samoa after the tsunami, contaminated water was a significant problem. Not only was it critical to remember never to drink from the faucet or use tap water while brushing teeth, but we also had to come up with creative solutions while seeing patients in the clinic and when cooking meals. It was hard to convince the Samoan children who love to swim that their favorite swimming beach was now off limits. It was always a priority to remind ourselves and the Pacific Islanders to stay hydrated, counteracting the effects of the hot, tropical climate. We returned home with a renewed sense of thanksgiving for our abundant supply of clean water.

Even water that has been treated and comes out of your tap can have contaminants that affect your health. Although your water supplier may be doing everything it can to provide you with safe tap water, chemicals can enter your water in your own home. Lead is one such contaminant[6] and is of particular concern for pregnant women and young children. Lead poisoning can damage the nervous system and brain. Although lead exposure is more common from paint and dust, lead can come from leaded pipe and solder in your home water system.

Animals and birds, as well as humans, contaminate water. You can get sick from drinking water from a creek even though the creek is way up in the mountains, far away from any regular human activity. Drinking contaminated water can introduce parasites to your body. Most of these cause gastrointestinal illness until treated, but some can affect the brain.[7]

You don't have to *drink* bad water to get sick. Recreational water illnesses, according to the US Centers for Disease Control and Prevention, are illnesses that are spread by swallowing, breathing, or having contact with contaminated water from swimming pools, spas, lakes, rivers, or oceans.[8] These infections can cause neurologic problems. Children, pregnant women, and people with compromised immune systems are more at risk if they acquire such an infection.

The EPA oversees the nation's standards for the quality of tap water when that water comes from a water supply other than a private well or spring. The regulations are enforced by most state environmental agencies. Since 1974, over eighty different contaminants have been regulated. Public water suppliers are required to provide an annual water quality report called a Consumer Confidence Report. This report tells you what contaminants are found in the water you drink, and whether they are found at levels that you should be concerned about.

SHARPER BRAIN TIPS

- Take dehydration seriously. Most Americans drink less water daily than they should.
- Realize that dehydration can contribute to a significant drop in performance.
- Remind older adults to drink water often during the day. They are more at risk for dehydration than people of other age groups.
- Don't spend your money on bottled water, if yours is from a municipal supply, unless you want to avoid exposure to all treatments of the water that may have occurred.
- Drink approximately one-half ounce of water per pound of your weight per day in order to stay properly hydrated (if you are not exercising or pregnant, in which case you need more).
- Recognize these signs of dehydration: dry mouth and lips, dizziness, rapid weight loss, confusion or change in mental state, reduced or concentrated urine.
- Don't overdo it. Too much water can leach essential nutrients from your system.
- Do not drink water from any natural source, unless you are absolutely sure it is safe.

31

Cardiphonia

With him I dare be free, and am not sorry, but glad, that . . . not a thought of my heart is hidden from him."
— John Newton[1]

DOWN THROUGH THE AGES, THEOLOGIANS AND MYSTICS HAVE tried to describe true spirituality and how to achieve it. Most often, they've peered within, probing the dance of their own souls with the supernatural in an effort to deepen their own spiritual lives. And they've written about this journey inward in order to help others learn to do the same, as John Newton did in *Cardiphonia*, which means "utterance of the heart."[2]

Many terms have been used to describe the process of becoming more spiritual, but the word "spirituality" did not come into existence until the 5th Century among the clergy, and it was not used in common speech until toward the end of the Middle Ages. Its root meaning comes from Genesis, which says that God breathed into Adam's nostrils the breath of life. Perhaps the search for God that is common among all humankind is like trying to follow the scent of God. To paraphrase one of our scientific friends: When God's spirit swirled and flowed through Adam's nasal passages, was Adam imprinted with the scent of

God? Is our spiritual quest as simple as learning to discern between things that smell of God and life versus things that smell of evil and death?[3]

Up until very recently, scientists could only speculate about such matters, since there was no way to quantify the metaphysical. But now, equipped with high tech scanners, the new science of "neuro-spirituality" is asking questions like: What is the relationship between the brain and the soul? How shall we even speak of the immaterial (soul, or mind, or God, for example) when we are studying the material, in this case, the brain and its functions?

This new scientific endeavor raises interesting questions like: "Will the soul show up in an MRI? And can you scan the brain and see exactly what parts are being activated during a particular practice, such as *lectio divina*? [the practice of Scriptural reading, meditation, and prayer intended to promote communion with God].[4] If so, will that be consistent from person to person? And does every [spiritual] practice activate a unique part of the brain?"[5]

Some scientists are making progress toward answering these types of questions. For example, for some time scientists have speculated about whether there is a "God spot" in the brain— one distinct area responsible for spirituality. One scientist claims to have found an answer: "We have found a neuropsychological basis for spirituality, but it's not isolated to one specific area of the brain," said Brick Johnstone, PhD. "Spirituality is a much more dynamic concept that uses many parts of the brain. Certain parts of the brain play more predominant roles, but they all work together to facilitate individuals' spiritual experiences."

Johnstone and his colleagues studied twenty people with traumatic brain injuries affecting the right parietal lobe, the area of the brain situated a few inches above the right ear. They surveyed participants on characteristics of spirituality, such as how close they felt to a higher power and if they felt their lives were part of a divine plan. They found that those with more significant injury to their right parietal lobe showed an increased feeling of closeness to a higher power. "Since our research shows that people with this impairment are more spiritual," Johnstone said, "this suggests spiritual experiences are associated with a decreased focus on the self. This is consistent with many religious texts that suggest people should concentrate on the wellbeing of others rather than on themselves."[6]

If spirituality relies on many parts of the brain working together, keeping your brain as healthy as possible is goal number one if you want to know God and be known by him as intimately as possible, which is the ultimate goal of any spiritual quest. Think of your spiritual life as a partnership. The Maker wants you to do your part in keeping the equipment he gave you in good working order. The Scriptures contain many guidelines for a healthy lifestyle which will help you reach your full potential as a human being. These guidelines involve more than just what you eat and drink. They encompass every aspect of living —physically, emotionally, relationally, and spiritually. When you are not whole in any of these, you are less than whole in all of them, and this has far reaching effects on your health in general, and on your brain's health in particular. This is why living a truly spiritual life is a complex endeavor, and not just something reserved for one day of the week.

For example, when your mind is torn apart by worry, you cannot expect your brain to function well or to rest well, if you provide it with the opportunity to rest at all. Or when your relationships are marked by turmoil and strife, your mind will be distressed, and this stress will affect your brain's health in many ways. Or if you are living on fast food and diet soda, you can hardly expect your brain to have the energy it needs in order to faithfully follow wherever the Spirit may lead.

Our Creator knows your weaknesses and will enable you to live a healthier, more spiritually productive life when you stop trying to do it all on your own and in your own way, and ask him to guide and empower you to follow the Manual. The magnificent brain he designed for you can be re-wired from worry to trust. You can learn to see problems as possibilities for deepening your relationship with God as you accept his love and forgiveness, which you can then extend to others. And as you feed your neurons well, you are following the apostle's advice that whatever you eat or drink, or whatever you do, you do it all to the glory of God (1 Corinthians 10:31).

Brain health expert Dr. Paul Nussbaum lists spirituality as one of the five components of brain health. "Spirituality encompasses more than an appreciation for religious values," Nussbaum says. "At its essence, it means for you to turn inward away from the material world and its hurried demands to a more peaceful existence. Spiritual practices can involve prayer, meditation . . . quiet contemplation, or any other relaxation that helps you slow down and connect with the essence of who you are and what you value in life. It can also be an effective way to fight stress."[7]

SHARPER BRAIN TIPS

- List three things in your life that affect your "spirituality."
- Think of the most "spiritual" person you've known and describe why you feel that way about him or her. What can you do today to emulate those characteristics?
- Use deep breathing exercises to help you relax. Feel the stress leave.
- Take a walk in a natural setting, letting your senses register everything you see, hear, smell, touch, or taste. Let these things remind you of the Creator. Draw close to him and he will draw close to you.
- Learn how to use techniques of Christian meditation, including asking God to help you to know how to pray, especially when you cannot find the words (see Romans 8:26).

32

Bug Off

The smallest insect may cause death by its bite.
– Ancient Proverb[1]

WHEN I (DAVE) WAS ABOUT SIXTEEN, I SERVED AS A COUNselor at a Christian camp not too far from my home in Vermont, where mosquitoes were more than just pests, though until then I never thought of them as mortal enemies. All counselors and campers were required to purchase a very inexpensive insurance policy, which most likely had to pay very few claims, since campers were there only a week at a time and our most risky contact sport was eating breakfast. But that year one camper had the misfortune of contracting "sleeping sickness" (equine encephalitis), which I had never heard about but have never forgotten since then.

As it turned out, the pool and the stream that fed it were producing an impressive crop of mosquitoes that year, one of which had evidently dined upon a nearby horse that was infected with the eastern equine encephalomyelitis (EEE) virus, before it selected that particular camper for dessert. Equine encephalitis is preventable in horses, but difficult to treat in humans, since there is no cure for the virus (about 35 percent of infected humans die from this illness). When the insurance company was forced to pay for that camper's care, there was much ado about it in the camp, where we all engaged in a massive mosquito control effort, including closing and treating the pool and putting the brook off limits to all but the trout.

Since then (the mid-1960s) several insect-borne diseases with potential central nervous system (CNS) consequences have burst on the scene, including Lyme disease (tick-borne, discovered 1975) and the West Nile virus (mosquito-borne, discovered 1999). These, added to Rocky Mountain Spotted fever (tick-borne, discovered in the 1930s) now provide anyone informed in these matters just cause to either stay inside when the temperature is above freezing, or to ensure that they, and everyone they care about, are well protected when they venture forth into the insect empire known as the great outdoors.

Lyme disease is spread by ticks with an affinity for whitetail deer. According to the CDC, this disease affects about 16,000 people per year in the US, mostly in the northeastern, mid-Atlantic, and upper north-central regions, and in several counties in northwestern California.[2] Though it is treatable, especially early on, many cases are not recognized either by the patient or the healthcare provider until it is possible that there may be long-term CNS (and other) effects. Many people have been fighting this infection for years—some, like our teacher-friend Patty, whose story follows, for more than thirty years, with significant ongoing health results.

Patty wrote: "Although Lyme disease can be cured, especially if caught right away, 20 percent of us continue to struggle for unknown reasons, with no end in sight. I wanted to defend myself by saying that I work a full-time job and a part-time job to pay my massive medical bills and for my meds, since the health insurance companies decided I was the equivalent of Typhoid Mary. I wanted to whine about having to sleep every second when it wasn't absolutely necessary to be dressed and upright. I wanted to cry about my messy house that is last on my 'What can I manage today?' list. I wanted to complain about the crippling fatigue that comes in spells, and discouragement over not being able to do simple things that others take for granted."

The West Nile virus (WNV), which is now a world-wide pandemic, is carried by mosquitoes that have (usually) ingested blood from infected birds. It was first identified in the Western Hemisphere in 1999, in and around New York City, when seven patients presented with similar symptoms, and all of them died. The primary evidence was sick and dying crows, of which there were more than 10,000 found. It is thought that the first infected bird was brought into the US illegally, but no one will ever know.

Extensive studies of donated blood have shown that approximately 1 percent of Americans have antibodies to WNV, meaning they have been infected at one time or another. The good news, if there is any, about WNV, is that most infected persons survive. In fact, most infected persons do not even know they have been infected.

The other good news is that for insect-borne diseases with CNS implications, prevention of infection can be the same for mosquitoes as it is for ticks. You can obtain some protection from your clothing—in fact, there are fine mesh suits available, complete with head nets. The most effective repellents contain DEET (N,N-diethyl-meta-toluamide), picaridin, oil of lemon eucalyptus, or IR 3535 (3-[N-Butyl-N-acetyl]-aminopropionic acid, ethyl ester), which is an active ingredient in at least one US-made product. This repellent has been used in Europe for more than twenty years with no adverse side effects. Scientists have recently developed a new insect repellent that is made from oil of catmint. This has been shown to be effective with mosquitoes. No information is available on its effectiveness against ticks, but if you choose this one your cat may love you to death.

Some of the most effective killers of human beings in history have been insects—mosquitoes, ticks, fleas, and such. From malaria to the plague, and everything between, the only way to avoid becoming infected is to be protected. Even if you are "green" (i.e. prefer natural products vs. manufactured products) in your overall lifestyle, being "mean" (using man-made repellants) may be more effective, especially when exposure to insects is prolonged.[3]

So the choice, especially for parents trying to protect their children, is a real dilemma—you must decide how to reduce the risk of illness from insects; and, you must weigh the benefits versus the risks of the various insecticides available. Do the research, but do not do nothing to protect yourself and those you love when you do spend time outdoors.

SHARPER BRAIN TIPS

- Stay inside at dawn and dusk if you can.
- Wear light colored long-sleeved shirts and light colored pants, tucked into your socks, if you want to avoid ticks. Some outdoor clothing contains a chemical that kills mosquitoes.
- Do not depend on supplements to make you less tasty to mosquitoes; scientific evidence is lacking to support such claims.
- Carefully examine new products—their claims and their safety—before using.
- Stay abreast of new options: I, Dave, had good success using a product called ThermaCELL to repel mosquitoes, even when I was out and about in the swampy areas of Florida. This works without touching the skin or clothing.
- Please: Take this chapter seriously; you could save yourself and those you love from a lifetime of suffering and grief.

33

You are Hard Wired for Joy

Rejoice in the Lord always. I will say it again: Rejoice!
– The Apostle Paul, from Prison
(Philippians 4:4, NIV)

Depending on which Bible translation you prefer, the word "rejoice" appears close to 300 times in the text. Its root concept is "joy," which is more than mere happiness, since happiness is connected to good happenings. Joy is a much more settled attitude of the soul, contributing to stable emotions, a sound mind, and a strong will committed to living a life of love for God and one's fellow men.

Modern technology's non-invasive probing of the human brain can actually show the positive effect that joy has on that organ. This data is worth considering even if one is not seeking a life of joy via the pathway of faith. For if sadness, depression, despair, and their associates cause disease in one's brain and joy and its associates create a context for optimal brain health, then it's a "no-brainer" for anyone interested in having the healthiest brain possible to find out all there is to know about this matter.

Thankfully, all there is to know on this matter is fairly simple. When we're sad, angry, afraid, anxious, or addicted to some person, place, thing, or activity—our brain shows it when examined using SPECT (single photon emission computed tomography). SPECT is "a nuclear medicine tomographic imaging technique using gamma rays. It is very similar to conventional nuclear medicine planar imaging using a gamma camera. However, it is able to provide true 3D information."[1] When we're content, hopeful, happy, and healthy (emotionally), the SPECT results show that, too. How it's done and how it's read are both book-length subjects, but one scientist investigating brain health using SPECT has written the book, *This Is Your Brain on Joy*.

Dr. Earl Henslin is a colleague of Dr. Daniel Amen—a pioneer in this field—whose SPECT scan work shows an individual's brain while he or she is reacting, not just at rest. By interpreting the areas that "light up" in a person's brain at certain times, doctors can gain insight about why some people are dysthymic (chronically mildly depressed or irritable), or have rage issues, or are obsessive-compulsives like the beloved TV character, "Monk," of the show by that name.

Dr. Henslin's SPECT scans reveal numerous details (not whether a particular brain is "normal," but which areas are more efficiently "wired" for a happy life). Interestingly enough, these brain scans reveal a sort of cerebral happy face if you concentrate on the illuminated sections of the brain while the patient is experiencing joy. Is this the Creator's sense of humor, to make our brains match our smiles when we are in the talons of joy?[2]

The researchers are looking at a variety of therapeutic options including psychotherapy, supplements, or prescription medications, sometimes all three, to see which can restore a particular patient to a happier state.

"What you choose to do, think about, surround yourself with, and put in your gullet make a difference," says Henslin. "It all matters to your experience of joy on this planet."[3] In addition, Henslin emphasizes that those who pray and meditate each day not only increase their peace and joy, but the calming effects of those two activities become more effective as time goes on, if they become a regular habit.[4]

In other words, even when times are tough, our choices about how and with whom to face adversity are perhaps the most important keys to rejoicing even in sorrow. Jesus, who was known as a man of sorrows, often spoke of joy. In one instance, he had just told his disciples of his coming death, and then he said: "I have told you this so that my joy may be in you and that your joy may be complete" (John 15:11, NIV).

Some people prefer psychotherapy, medications, supplements, scented candles, soft music, or any number of non-religious means to try to build a bridge to joy. Our recommendation is to use all the proven means available, including faith-related means, since with this approach you have nothing to lose and everything to gain, including something Jesus described as a joy that no one can take away.

SHARPER BRAIN TIPS

- If you are a person of faith, consider the implications of Psalm 16:11: "In Your presence is fullness of joy; in Your right hand are pleasures forever" (NASB).
- Send yourself some flowers, with a thank you note . . . for something you did for someone else.
- Ask yourself: What color is joy? Choose something that color and wear it today.
- Bite the freshest, sweetest, crunchiest apple you can, and savor the taste for thirty seconds.
- Hide a note that expresses hope in a corked bottle, and leave it for someone (anyone) to find.
- Create a treasure hunt for your kids, or neighborhood kids, and share their joy as they hunt.
- Play with a puppy, kitten, or child. Let their free-flowing joy invade your soul.

34

Where Past and Future Meet

To look backward for awhile is to refresh the eye, to restore it, and to render it the more fit for its prime function of looking forward.   – *Margaret Fairless Barber*[1]

HAVE YOU EVER BEEN IN THE MIDDLE OF DOING SOMETHING when all of a sudden something happens that triggers a memory, and you are beamed back into a past event that is as clear to you as though you were currently there? The feeling of nostalgia sweeps over you so intensely that you feel you are actually reliving the moment. It could be something as simple as a song you hear on the radio, a smell that reminds you of your grandmother's apple pie, a picture you see of the ocean at sunset that reminds you of a past romantic encounter, or something else equally mesmerizing, and you're suddenly off on a trip down memory lane.

Nostalgic memories usually replay pleasant events, which is why nostalgia can help when you are lonely, depressed, psychologically vulnerable, or threatened. Nostalgia is almost always associated with positive emotions even when the trigger is something negative. The memory can even be bittersweet (happiness mixed with sadness), but the mind will often juxtapose positive and negative elements to create redemption, moving the negative memory toward a positive one.

The research of Sedikides and others focuses on the positive and potentially therapeutic aspects of nostalgia. Their research suggests that "Nostalgia can promote psychological health by producing positive feelings, higher self-esteem, and an increase in the feeling of being loved and protected by others. Nostalgia may boost optimism, spark inspiration, and foster creativity. Nostalgia also counteracts effects of loneliness, by increasing perceptions of social support. Loneliness can also trigger nostalgia and this has important implications for the elderly who are vulnerable to social isolation. Nostalgia may actually help them overcome feelings of loneliness."[2]

Nostalgia is about storytelling—stories created and stored as memories in your brain. You've probably noticed that each time you remember a positive past event, person, or place, the details are a little different. This is because a particular memory is not "retrieved," but is, in essence, re-created each time you recall it, by a series of complex neural interactions. You've probably also noticed that as you grow older, the details of a particular event are fuzzier each time you recall it. This is again due to your brain re-creating, rather than retrieving, that particular story.[3]

Nostalgia provides a link between our past and present stories. By providing a positive view of the past, nostalgia serves to bring a greater sense of constructive continuity and meaning to our lives. While day-to-day living can become tedious and sometimes depressing, a positive look back at our own journey can change that perspective and add new meaning to what we are doing today.[4]

Nostalgia can create feelings of connection, because it isn't just about ourselves, but is also about our relationships with others. This creates a social context that helps us feel close to others who are important to us, and to feel that we are important to them, too.

Nostalgia can also help us place ourselves in the context of the history of our community—of course this assumes that we still live in or near the community of our upbringing. Visiting local museums is a great place to remember the history of our town, still being written through us. Old photographs help us see what our town (and the people in it) looked like "back in the olden days" when people walked to work, went to church, wore their Easter bonnets in the Easter Parade, and made their own clothes instead of paying someone a half-world away to do that. Another good source for nostalgic local information or photos is your local library, which is likely to have a section devoted to local history.

Scrapbooking is another way to preserve your most precious memories, for yourself and posterity. And with the advent of the digital age, a number of new methods exist that make it much easier to achieve a similar effect, as in "scrapbooking" online, or creating screensavers or a slideshow of your favorite photos, including nostalgic ones, on your computer screen whenever it's turned on.

However you practice your own nostalgic moments, keep in mind that old adage, "Nostalgia ain't what it used to be." No. It's even better!

SHARPER BRAIN TIPS

- Invite some long-time friends over for dessert and games, and play "I Remember When. . . ." Give each person a 3x5 card when they arrive, with just those words written on it. Then listen, laugh, maybe cry, but definitely connect as each person who wants to share does so.

- Have a family hymn-sing, with participants singing various parts (if your family is musically inclined). Dave's family did this as part of the family's weekend celebration of his parents' sixtieth wedding anniversary. "It's amazing how easily those hymns flooded our minds and warmed our hearts," Dave recalls. "It wasn't exactly 'Daddy sang bass; Momma sang tenor,' but it was close."

- As part of your personal devotions, each day for one month write down a single sentence that connects you and a particular memory with special spiritual significance. At the end of the month, read them all back to yourself, out loud, and then thank God for his love, grace, and kindness to treat you this way.

- Make a "voice quilt" for special anniversaries, birthdays, and so forth. One family created voice quilts to honor their parents' eightieth birthdays, inviting a host of family and friends to contribute. The process is simple: Participants receive a telephone number to call, where they can record their comments. Many shared greetings began with "remember when." In the process of listening to these, a myriad of faded memories resurfaced, and the neurological connections were renewed. Now that's a synaptic event for sure.

- Go through the family album, reminiscing with at one other person as you turn the pages.

35

Buoy Your Amygdala

The sky is falling! The sky is falling!   – Chicken Little

E MOTIONS SUCH AS WORRY, FEAR, GUILT, ANXIETY, AND ANGER are hazardous to your health. Scientists have known for years that these and other emotions can cause a myriad of physical problems, and are the culprits behind many mental and emotional problems, such as depression, anxiety, and panic disorders.

In recent years studies have shown just how damaging these emotions can be to your brain health, and the research is showing that if you want your brain to be happy, you need to be happy, too. One of the ways to be happy is to take control of your emotions instead of allowing them to control you.

New York neuroscientist Joseph Ledoux has studied how the brain processes emotions, especially fear. He describes the "Amygdala, the almond-shaped brain structure that interprets emotion, as 'the hub in the brain's wheel of fear.' When the amygdala is stimulated, there is an outpouring of stress hormones, causing a state of hyper-vigilance. The amygdala processes the primitive emotions of fear, hate, love, bravery, and anger—all neighbors in the deep limbic brain. When the amygdala malfunctions, a mood disorder, or state of uncontrollable apprehension results." The amygdala, then, is an important component of the circuit that regulates negative emotion.[1]

This is further explained by Timothy Stokes, PhD: "[The amygdala] plays a central role in the storage of 'emotion memories'—unconscious memories of past hurts: times, especially in childhood, when we were painfully rejected, physically harmed, humiliated, helplessly frustrated, and so on. An emotion memory is recalled unconsciously. These memories are very durable and without intervention they may last a long time—even a lifetime. These emotion memories create feelings that are not appropriate to our immediate situation. When an emotion memory is active, we make distorted assumptions about our current situation. Hormones inhibit the reality-testing part of our brain, leading us to believe and even defend a distorted view of what is going on."[2] Unfortunately, these problems are being generated by brains that are functioning exactly as they were designed to function.

Fear is the underlying and primary emotion for much of what we feel and how we behave. It's part of our genetic makeup and functions to keep us safe in dangerous situations. You may be familiar with the "fight or flight" response to stimuli. When confronted with a situation that we are unfamiliar with or afraid of, all of our bodily systems are sent into a state of hyper alertness. The result is an outpouring of hormones, including adrenaline, followed by the steroid hormone cortisol. This helps us to quickly assess the situation and whether we need to flee or fight. If we hear a strange noise in our home at night, our senses shift into alert mode and we will either go investigate or decide that it's nothing. We can call 911 or calm down.[3]

When there is something stressful or fearful that we need to deal with, we have an adrenaline rush. The problem comes when stress becomes constant, rather than transitory. The result is worry, anxiety, and even panic. Panic is a heightened state of anxiety. Anxiety, distress, panic, and fear are closely related negative emotional states associated with physical or psychological harm. Anxiety is characterized by the anticipation of being harmed in the future, whereas fear is the anticipation of being harmed in the present. Distress is characterized by the awareness of being harmed at this particular moment. All of these can diffuse into one harmful emotional state or another.[4]

Bob was a consummate worrier. He worried about his job, being able to care for his family, having enough money to pay his bills, his health, and just about everything else. A child of the Depression, he grew up without enough and this mindset stayed with him the rest of his life. Even after receiving a rather large inheritance and investing it wisely, he worried about outliving his savings. His wife told him not to worry, that God would take care of them.

Bob did without many comforts through the years because of his fear that he wouldn't have enough. He didn't outlive his savings and left his widow comfortable, although not wealthy. She has now picked up his mantle of worry and is concerned that she will outlive her savings, although she is very frugal and has done well. She is learning, however, that all of this worry and fear could shorten her life and she is doing some of the things she always wanted to do, such as travel, trusting that God will indeed provide—just as he always has.

SHARPER BRAIN TIPS

- Try to recall the most distressing thing you were worried about one year ago today. Has that concern been resolved?

- If you have a major concern now that is draining you, take a "Google Map" approach and "zoom out" your perspective. Does your concern seem as worrisome from 30,000 feet—as in an airplane? From the moon—as in being an astronaut?

- Make a list of ten things you could do, right now, about this particular concern. These can range from outrageous (e.g. hire a clown to take your mind off the issue) to what a lot of people do (e.g. nothing), to anything in between. From this list, choose the most constructive and responsible course of action. Do that until it succeeds or fails. If it fails, lather, rinse, and repeat until you run out of ideas. Then start over.

- Each day, write down what worries you most at that moment. Create a "worry box," in which you place these notes. At some regular interval (monthly, quarterly, annually) empty the box and review the lists. Then make a new list of only the ones that are still a source of anxiety and put that list back into the box. Shred the others.

- Remember the Swedish proverb, "Worry often gives a small thing a big shadow."

- Remember the words of Jesus, "Therefore do not be anxious about tomorrow, for tomorrow will be anxious for itself. Sufficient for the day is its own trouble" (Matthew 6:34, ESV).

- Visualize a stop sign and call it to mind when you start to go down a rabbit trail of worry or fear. Your amygdala will thank you.

36

The Secret of Your Senses

When you start using senses you've neglected, your reward is to see the world with completely fresh eyes.
  — Barbara Sher, career counselor, author[1]

Imagine going through life without the ability to see the beauty around you, taste your favorite foods, smell your world after a spring rain, touch those you love, or to hear your favorite sounds. If you didn't have your senses, your world would be a very boring, and even unsafe, place.

Those of us who have our senses in working order, that is the senses of sight, taste, smell, touch, hearing, and often forgotten number six, proprioception (defined below), tend to take them for granted until they become less acute as we age. Scientists have long known that as we grow older, the way our senses transmit information about our world changes. These changes happen slowly over the course of aging so that we often don't notice subtle decreases, especially with the sense of smell, taste, and touch. The most dramatic changes occur with vision and hearing.

Our senses receive information from the environment, such as light and sound vibrations. Receptors in our sense organs convert this information into nerve impulses which are then carried to the brain. Our brains interpret these impulses into the correct sensation. We require a certain amount of stimulation before a sensation is perceived. This is a minimum level or a "threshold." Aging increases the threshold so that the amount of sensory input necessary to be aware of the sensation becomes greater.[2]

The following is a brief description of six of your senses, how they change as you age and what you can do to help keep them young:

> **Hearing:** Your ears have two jobs—hearing and helping you to maintain balance. As you age, your ear structures deteriorate. The eardrum may thicken and the inner ear bones and other structures are affected. It often becomes more difficult to maintain balance. There may be hearing loss, especially for high-frequency sounds. The sharpness of hearing starts declining after the age of fifty. Your brain may have a decreased ability to process sounds into meaningful information. Some people with significant hearing loss may require hearing aids.
>
> What can you do? Turn down the music, but keep listening. Music is a great brain stimulant. Combining sensory stimulation helps build new associations between areas of the brain. Try watching a sport in which you know the rules and the meaning of the referee's or umpire's signals on TV with the volume muted. For example, you might watch Monday Night Football to a CD of waltzes by Johann Strauss II.[3]
>
> **Vision:** Age-related changes in vision can occur as early as your thirties. Fewer tears will be produced and your eyes will be drier. As you age, the sharpness of your vision gradually declines and cataracts may begin to form. There are also changes in response to darkness or bright light, thus the inability of some seniors to drive at night. Corrective eyewear will help with most of the

problems you incur as you age. Your peripheral vision will decrease, making it harder to drive and do other activities you've enjoyed. In addition, your ability to distinguish colors decreases. It becomes harder to distinguish blues and greens than reds and yellow.[4]

What can you do? Have a yearly eye exam to make sure that any deterioration of vision is due to normal aging. Keep your eyes active with reading and other activities that help keep your vision sharp and stimulate your brain.

Taste and Smell: The senses of taste and smell are closely related. Most taste comes from odors. In addition to providing enjoyment, these senses alert us to dangers such as spoiled food, hazardous materials, and smoke. You have approximately 9,000 taste buds. Their number starts decreasing around the age of forty to fifty in women and fifty to sixty in men. Sensitivity to salty, sweet, bitter, and sour tastes doesn't decrease until after age sixty. The sense of smell usually doesn't diminish until after age seventy.

What can you do? Try new foods, such as ethnic foods, that use a variety of herbs and spices, which will stimulate your sense of taste and smell. Change your menu to add variety and new tastes and smells. Try aromatherapy and enjoy a wide range of smells.

Touch: When you touch something your brain interprets the type and amount of sensation. It also interprets the sensation as pleasant or unpleasant. Many studies have shown that with aging, you may have reduced or changed sensations of pain, vibration, cold, heat, pressure, and touch. It may be that some of the normal changes of aging are caused by decreased blood flow to the touch receptors or to the brain and spinal cord. The increasing inability to discern between temperatures, vibration, touch, pressure, and decreased sensitivity to pain can increase risk of injuries.

What can you do? Dig in your garden with your hands, try a pottery class, make cookies and mix the dough with your hands, gently caress your spouse's neck (or add massage to your intimate times together), stroke your cat until it purrs, try to catch your goldfish without looking into the bowl—any activity that keeps those touch receptors and your brain alive and well.

Proprioception: This is often referred to as our sixth sense and is critically important to our everyday function even though it is so unconscious that few even know it is there. "Proprioception refers to the brain's ability to know where our body is in space. The brain gathers information from a wide range of senses and then processes this information in order to compare it with a virtual body map . . . stored in our memory."[5] Without this important sense we might walk into door frames, bump into people as we pass them on the sidewalk or in a crowded room, and not be able to judge how close we are coming to the curb as we drive. This sense allows us to generate and maintain our upright posture and physical balance. If our body-in-space sense is diminished we must tune up all our other senses to compensate, which can lead to tiredness or loss of concentration.

What can you do? Try activities that challenge your balance like balancing on a wobble board in the gym or taking a Pilates class.

SHARPER BRAIN TIPS

- For hearing, combine sensory stimulation from sound with one or more other senses.
- For vision, throughout the day, alternate between looking at things that are near or far away.
- For taste and smell, for one week vary your foods, and from time to time compare how the food tastes while holding your nose.
- For touch, have someone set objects with differing shapes and textures on a table, then try to identify them using only your hands and your eyes closed or blindfolded.
- For proprioception (knowing where your body is in space), when standing outdoors or in a large room, try to estimate distances between various objects and your right foot.

37

Synaptic Serenades

Music produces a kind of pleasure which human nature cannot do without.
— *Confucius*

YOU DON'T HAVE TO BE A GENIUS TO KNOW THAT LISTENING to good music is good for you. But it helps. Einstein said, "If I were not a physicist, I would probably be a musician. I often think in music. I live my daydreams in music. I see my life in terms of music."

Perhaps you know these words from the old hymn, "This is my Father's world, and to my listening ears all nature sings, and round me rings the music of the spheres." In a very real sense, music is the universal language. This may be one reason that almost everyone, including Einstein, would admit that music has had a profound effect in their lives, from making them laugh, cry, relive old memories, love others, to helping them heal emotionally, and maybe even physically, from life's wounds, and so on.

Music is, without question, one of our Creator's greatest gifts to humankind. And the many examples of worship with songs, instruments, and dance in the Scriptures depict ways in which we can use that gift to worship him.

But music is not just good for the soul; it is good for your body and mind.

Neurologist and author, Dr. Oliver Sacks said, "All of us have all sorts of personal experiences with music. We find ourselves calmed by it, excited by it, comforted by it, mystified by it and often haunted by it. It can lift us out of depression or move us to tears. I am no different. I need music to start the day and as company when I drive. I need it when I go for swims and runs. I need it, finally, to still my thoughts when I retire, to usher me into the world of dreams."[1]

Science has long known the benefits of music physically and psychologically. Daniel Levitin, a psychologist who studies the neuroscience of music at McGill University in Montreal, wrote, in *This is Your Brain on Music*, "Music listening and music therapy have been shown to help people overcome a broad range of psychological and physical problems."[2]

Scientists are just beginning to know why these benefits occur by studying the effects that music has on the brain itself. Cognitive neuroscience of music is the scientific study of brain-based mechanisms involved in the cognitive processes underlying music. An early study by the University of Texas determined that music is perceived in many areas of the brain. For example, melody is processed on the right side of the brain, while lyrics are understood on the left side of the brain in areas that process language. Rhythm is processed in several different areas of the brain.[3]

In the ensuing years since that study, scientists have been better able to identify areas of the brain that are responsible for music listening, composing, performing, reading, writing, and what parts of the brain are involved in music "emotions," relying on direct observation of the brain through such techniques as fMRIs, EEGs, and so on. One effect that has showed up in many studies is that listening to music releases dopamine in your brain, which is a key to feeling more pleasure and less pain.[4]

Dr. Oliver Sacks has studied the effect of music on the neurologically impaired and reports that, "For reasons we do not yet understand, musical abilities often are among the last to be lost, even in cases of widespread brain damage." Someone who is disabled by a stroke or by Alzheimer's or another form of dementia may still be able to respond to music. Sacks said there is promise that some of these patients may regain the ability to carry out certain tasks when the prompts are put in the form of a verse or song, such as "'One, two, buckle my shoe.'"[5]

Stephan, a songwriter, reports that he has in the past spent a lot of time in nursing homes playing for the patients there. "I clearly remember one woman who was always slumped over in her wheel chair, not really connecting with what was going on or saying anything . . . until I started playing hymns. Then, she lifted her head, sat up in her chair, and sang every word of those songs. When the music was over, she went back into her own world.

A recent article describes how participants who were about to undergo surgery were randomly assigned to either take anti-anxiety drugs or listen to music. The patients who listened to music had less anxiety and lower cortisol than people who took drugs. "The promise here is that music is arguably less expensive than drugs, and it's easier on the body and it doesn't have side effects," author Dr. Daniel Levitin said.[6]

SHARPER BRAIN TIPS

- Make music part of your everyday life—listen while driving, exercising, doing chores, while falling asleep, and as a friend posted on Facebook—"Cooking to music is always so much more fun."
- De-stress yourself by putting on headphones, lying back comfortably, and becoming part of the music.
- If you have young children or grandchildren, help them develop a love of music.
- Join a choir, perhaps at your church, or in your community. That way your enjoyment compounds—unless you can't carry a tune in a bucket.
- Sing, because to sing alone is recreation; to sing together is jubilation.

38

De-myth-ti-fying Brain Health

Age is an issue of mind over matter. If you don't mind, it doesn't matter. – Mark Twain

BEFORE YOU READ THIS CHAPTER, TAKE THE FOLLOWING QUIZ. Mark each statement T or F (for True or False):

1. ___ I only use 10 percent of my brain.
2. ___ If my brain cells are injured or die, they cannot be replaced.
3. ___ Working my brain nonstop will boost my brain power.
4. ___ My likelihood of developing Alzheimer's is controlled by my genes.
5. ___ I was born with all the brain cells I'll ever have.
6. ___ I can permanently increase my IQ by using cognitive training programs.

7. ___ Decline of brain function is inevitable as you age.
8. ___ Listening to Mozart will make me smarter.
9. ___ Supplements will improve my brain health.

We could print the answers upside down somewhere, but they are all: FALSE.

Now let's consider them one by one:

MYTH #1
Human beings only use 10 percent of their brains.

Though it's impossible to trace the origin of this myth, advertisers have made ample use of the concept by suggesting that buying a certain product or book, or the use of some program or device, can tap your alleged great reservoir of unused brain power. Some time ago, for example, ABC television advertised their program "The Secret Lives of Men" with the blurb: "Men only use ten percent of their brains."

Brain scanning has shown that our brains are always active. It's just that some areas are active at one time (say while we're threading a needle) while other areas are relatively inactive as we focus on the task. In a normal day, your entire brain (unless some area has been damaged) gets a workout . . . to the degree that you engage in neuronal exercise.

MYTH #2
Brain cells that are injured or die cannot be replaced.

We all know people who have experienced brain injuries and then regained their faculties. The human brain is far more resilient than was once thought. In fact, surgeries are sometimes done to remove half the brain of people with serious neurological disorders, with no effect on personality of memory.[1]

Like other cells in the body, brain cells die . . . at a rate of about 1,500 per day. But these cells are replaced. And research is showing that the total of new neurons produced (for example, in the hippocampus) can be increased through choices to learn, live a healthier lifestyle, reduce stress, get enough rest, and so forth. One program that specializes in this result is The Neurology Institute for Brain and Fitness.[2]

MYTH #3
Working my brain nonstop will boost your brain power.

Your heart works nonstop, at first glance. But even your heart rests between beats. The old archery proverb applies: "The bow that is always bent will break." According to the Franklin Institute, "As science gains greater insight into the consequences of stress on the brain, the picture that emerges is not a pretty one. A chronic overreaction to stress overloads the brain with powerful hormones that are intended only for short-term duty in emergency situations. Their cumulative effect damages and kills brain cells."[3]

You may be tempted to multi-task to get more done, but your brain really wants to focus on one thing at a time. This conflict invites inefficiency and added stress, while focusing on one thing at time, even for a short time, will accomplish more. Try this sometime: Instead of trying to focus on four things that keep going round and round in your mind, focus on one of them for fifteen minutes, then the next, and the next until you're done. See if your efficiency and effectiveness both benefit.

MYTH #4
Your genes determine your fate in terms of Alzheimer's.

While a person may be genetically predisposed to developing early-onset Alzheimer's (5 percent of Alzheimer's cases fit this description) there are genetic tests for this, and you might benefit from the results if early onset Alzheimer's (age 30-60 onset) is common in your family. In addition, research is identifying other genetic risk factors, but no one knows who some who are at greater risk, genetically speaking, actually do develop late-onset (after age 60) Alzheimer's. Genetic testing is not recommended for these risk factors, because the most common gene is present in 25 to 30 percent of the general population (and only 40 percent of those who actually develop Alzheimer's) so the potential anxiety of knowing you are even a little more at risk than others outweighs the benefit of that knowledge.[4]

These things having been said, about 85 percent of Alzheimer's cases have no genetic component. So practicing the healthy brain principles in this book—consume a brain-friendly diet, exercise, avoid substance abuse and exposure to toxins, get enough rest, reduce your stress, increase your social connections, challenge your mind with new things, and keep yourself healthy spiritually—will all keep your brain healthy and combat decline.

MYTH #5
You were born with all the brain cells you'll ever have.

Most people are born with about 100 billion brain cells. Until about the middle of the 20th Century, it was generally accepted among neuroscientists that the adult brain could not generate new cells. But a groundbreaking study caused a revision of the textbooks by demonstrating that brain cells can regenerate, thus opening a whole new field of scientific investigation that still continues today. While some scientists still doubt this assertion, evidence is mounting that keeping your mind active and engaged throughout life does protect you from the mental decline that often occurs in those whose lifestyle is more passive.

Physical exercise is one key, in that it increases a protein called brain-derived neurotropic factor (BDNF), which plays a role in the plasticity of brain cells as well as their survival and function. Other lifestyle elements—diet, rest, etc.—provide a healthy context in which these new cells may be produced.[5]

MYTH #6
When you were born, your IQ was set for life.

Most likely when you were in school you took an IQ (intelligence quotient) test, once, and that was it. About 95 percent of the population scores between 70 and 130; 100 is average. Although your IQ is one predictor of success in education and work, it is possible that vocational counselors have relied too much on this score in the past, because studies have shown that one's IQ score can fluctuate, and a lower than expected score might indicate a person was having a bad brain day.

With cognitive training, IQ scores can increase temporarily. This may be due in part to increased familiarity with the tests or the testing process as a result of multiple testings. *The Wall Street Journal* reported that, "Scores can change gradually or quickly, after as little as a few weeks of cognitive training, research shows. The increases are usually so incremental that they're not immediately perceptible to individuals, and the intelligence-boosting effects of cognitive training can fade after a few months."[6]

MYTH #7
Decline of brain function is inevitable as you age.

What you know based on experience remains stable as you age, but "fluid intelligence"—cognitive abilities not related to experience or education (such as decision making or adapting to, or learning new information quickly) may decline.

Your long-term memories will most likely stay with you, while more recent memories may be at risk. Your ability to focus may be better than some young folks, but it may be more difficult to do two things at the same time (for example, watch TV and talk on the phone). You will most likely retain your general verbal skills (though it may become more difficult to think of the precise word you want to use, or to remember people's names) and your problem solving will be based on accumulated wisdom and experience, which means that you may be good at resolving issues you've faced before, but need more time to deal with questions or situations that are new to you.[7]

You can retain your sharpness longer by practicing a healthy brain lifestyle: reduce stress, get enough rest, consume a healthy diet, stay engaged socially, keep your mind active, practice your faith.

MYTH #8
Listening to classical music will make you smarter.

In the early 1990s, a study was conducted at UC Irvine, in which teenage students were exposed to Mozart's "Sonata for Two Pianos in D Major." It was reported that these students performed better on reasoning tests that those who did not listen to the same piece. These results spawned a whole new industry promoting "The Mozart Effect." Even though other studies have shown this claim to be flawed, the myth survives. Listening to music can be better from your brain than not listening to music, but the effect is the same whether the music is classical or country.[8]

MYTH #9
Supplements will improve your brain health.

You've probably heard something like, "I took ginko biloba for three months and it made me smarter and sharper." This is anecdotal not scientific evidence. Or maybe you've heard, "Studies have shown that such and such does this or that, and the product we want you to buy contains such and such, so you can expect that our product will accomplish a similar result for you." To support a claim scientifically, a scientific study must be done on the specific product being described, not just one of its components, since other components in the same product may nullify or even negatively affect the expected outcome.

Good science is based on a "gold standard," which requires double-blind, placebo controlled, randomized trials conducted by independent/objective researchers.[9] Very little truly scientific evidence exists to support that any supplements will improve your brain health. Though such studies may be done in the future, it is unlikely that any company smaller than a pharmaceutical company could afford the costs involved.

SHARPER BRAIN TIPS

Agree/Disagree:

___ It's time to try to improve my IQ.

___ I plan to add brain games to my list of brain exercises, but I'll stick to free ones.

___ I will discover and practice everything that might keep my mind sharper.

___ I believe in the "Mozart Effect" and plan to continue listening to classical music for my brain's sake.

___ Since no one knows the effects of supplements on brain health, I am going to continue taking "brain health" supplements, because future studies may show that they actually work.

___ I'm going to give my mind a break on a regular basis, because it needs to rest, too.

___ I am going to carefully examine the truth of all brain gain claims I encounter.

39

Which Planet are *You* From?

Not only do men and women communicate differently but they think, feel, perceive, react, respond, love, need, and appreciate differently. They almost seem to be from different planets. . . ."
— *John Gray*[1]

QUESTION: IF MEN AND WOMEN THINK AND BEHAVE SO differently, does this come from their nature or their nurture? Answer: Yes.

On the one hand, with the exception of reproductive cells, every cell in the bodies of men and women differ in that women have two "X" chromosomes and men have one "X" and one "Y" chromosome. This includes brain cells. This is nature.

On the other hand, patterns of thought and behavior are affected to some degree by nurture; including many aspects of environment from upbringing to education to role models to personal experience.

Differences in males and female brains exist at every level from the smallest cell to the large structures, including a person's anatomy, physiology, chemical, and hormonal make up. It is not hard to imagine how this impacts everything from emotions and thinking to behavior. Studies indicate that key parts of the brain are different in size in males versus females. "Male brains contain 6.5 times more gray matter—the "thinking matter"—female brains have more than 9.5 times as much white matter—the "processing matter."[2]

In *His Brain – Her Brain*, Barb Larimore explains, "Understanding this can be critical in understanding our husbands—their stick-to-itiveness, steadfastness, determination, and single-mindedness. It also can assist their understanding and appreciation of us—our intuition and the way we can read people."[3]

Chemically, male and female brains are bathed in different hormones, starting before birth. Over seventy different chemicals act upon the brain in unique ways all through life. The way the brain is wired is also uniquely different. When we consider all the differences, it makes sense to wonder how we can relate to each other at all!

The title of the book *Men are From Mars, Women are From Venus* suggests (tongue-in-cheek) that men and women are so different they must be from different planets, so respecting each other's differences is crucial to establishing better relationships between the sexes, whether at home or at work. Many people have used the principles of that book to improve their understanding of and tolerance of male-female differences that might otherwise cause significant interpersonal conflict.

When you affirm that our Creator made us this way for good reasons, however, you open up a whole new perspective—the possibility of *celebrating and harnessing the power* of male-female differences at home and work.

A key part of the brain that is basic to the way we behave is the limbic system that controls our emotional responses and memory. For instance, the amygdala, which processes fear and action is wired differently and very often triggers opposite reactions in males and females. Males usually respond with a fight or flight mode and are programmed to want to be left alone and take action. However the female tendency will be the "tend or befriend" response and she will want to talk to her husband or girlfriend for reassurance and comfort.

Bestselling author, psychiatrist Daniel G. Amen, MD, has identified many differences in the brain activity of men and women, using single photon emission computed tomography (SPECT). "We compared the scans of 46,000 male and female brains using a study called SPECT, which looks at the blood flow and activity patterns," Dr. Amen said. "Out of eighty areas tested, females were significantly more active in seventy.... These differences help us understand some of the unique strengths and vulnerabilities of the female brain and give us important clues how to optimize it."

He explained, "Because of the increased activity, females often exhibit greater strengths in the areas of: empathy; intuition, or knowing something that is true without knowing exactly why; collaboration, which is why women often make better bosses; self-control, which is the reason why females go to jail dramatically less often than males; and appropriate worry.... But this increased activity also makes females more vulnerable to: anxiety; depression, which they suffer from twice as much as men; insomnia; eating disorders; pain; and being unable to turn off their thoughts."[4]

What might this look like in a marriage? The busy female brain allows her to multitask more often and to recognize subtle details. The male brain is more focused; often concentrating on providing, protecting, and conquering. It seems that, from the perspective of brain function, God's design for marriage is for each couple, together, to form a more "perfect whole." Yes, men and women may be "worlds apart" in some ways, but a couple's strengths and weaknesses often mirror each other. This allows them to handle situations in a unified and complete manner.

Two brains working together do a better job than one.

This is often revealed most vividly in emergency situations as we see in the Larimore's story about their son's accident one Easter Sunday as they were preparing dinner: Walt relates, "We heard a crash, then a scream, and a cry for help . . . my medical training kicked in. I rushed to Scott's side and quickly examined the wound. . . . I put pressure on the wound with my hand and called to Barb 'get a towel! We need to get to the ER' I turned to reassure my son he was going to be OK."

Barb adds her perspective, "After grabbing a clean towel for Walt, I told Kate to get in the car, called a friend to activate our church's prayer chain, turned off the oven, sprinkled cleanser on the blood on the floor, and locked the front door. After Walt carried Scott to the car, we drove to the ER. As Walt took care of Scott in an exam room, I kept Kate occupied, filled out forms, called my mom, and then planned how to would finish cooking dinner."[5]

The Creation story (Genesis 1) describes how God made everything and pronounced his handiwork "good," but after he made humankind as male and female (with all their differences) and made them stewards over everything else, he called what he had just done VERY GOOD. And so it is.

SHARPER BRAIN TIPS

- Learn all you can about your own brain and its unique way of functioning.
- Learn all you can about your spouse's (or significant other's) brain and its unique way of functioning.
- Embrace and celebrate the differences, and seek to harness their collaborative power.
- Become a student of your friends and family to discern their usual ways of interacting with the world as well as with you. Accept and honor their differences.
- Remember that his brain needs respect; hers needs love.

40

Unfoggin' Your Noggin

The brain is a wonderful organ. It starts working for you when you get up in the morning and doesn't stop until you get to the office.   – Robert Frost[1]

BRAIN FOG IS A COMMON CONDITION THAT MOST PEOPLE EXperience from time to time, but for which there is no clear-cut diagnosis, treatment, or clinical research available. If you were to ask ten people randomly encountered on the street if they had ever experienced brain fog, several if not most of them would say they had, though they might describe the experience differently. For example, they might say they felt: "sluggish," like they were "functioning in slow motion," "cloudy," "unfocused," "out of it," "spaced out," like they were "walking around in a dream," or "in a daze."

The main symptom of brain fog is lack of mental clarity, hence the use of the word, "fog," as in a low-flying cloud that hinders one's ability to see clearly. One online medical dictionary describes it as: A condition that affects all ages and which is characterized by confusion, decreased clarity of thought, and forgetfulness. It can lead to minor depression and, per some, crime and delinquency.

Despite its frequency, it is not regarded as a 'real' condition. Brain fog can be triggered by physical, psychological and per some, biochemical and spiritual factors including, allegedly, adrenal exhaustion, food and chemical reactions, nutritional deficiencies, stress, depression, or denial.[2]

Since the early 1800s, "clouding of consciousness" has been the standard term used for brain fog, though in today's psychiatric diagnostic and statistical manual of mental disorders (DSM-5) if falls into the category: "cognitive disorder not otherwise specified."

Quite often when middle-aged patients describe brain fog to their physician, they are worried that not being able to remember where they left their keys is an early sign of Alzheimer's or dementia setting in. In such cases, a wise doctor might suggest that forgetting where you left your keys is one thing, but forgetting how to use those keys is an entirely different matter.

Have any of these things happened to you?

- You leave the shopping list at home because it only has three things on it, but when you get to the store, you can't remember them.
- Then you go out to the parking lot and can't recall where you parked.
- You want to call your spouse, but can't recall the right cell phone number.
- You're trying to get ready for work, but can't seem to make yourself move fast enough.
- You're on your way somewhere and suddenly remember that you left the stove on.
- For a frightening thirty to ninety seconds, you can't remember where you are.

With brain fog, your awareness of yourself and your environment is diminished, as Patty's story clearly shows:

I'd swing the other foot down and sleep like that, both feet on the floor with my upper half still wrapped in the comforter. By the third buzz I would consider smashing the alarm clock but would pray instead, asking God why it was so all-fired important for me to get up. When he reminded me that I was a teacher, I would crawl out into the sunlight like a sailor with a hangover. That led to a comatose shower, sometimes donning my blouses inside out and great panic as I searched for my pocketbook.

My "terminal as an artist, I'd been told I was "weird" from a very young age, so most people never noticed when brain fog crept into my life. I knew it was blurring my thinking, unlike some Lyme patients who have terrifying spells where they can't recognize their husbands. Mercifully, my fuzziness was more benign. Mornings were particularly foggy. I would fit the snooze button and swing one foot over the edge of the bed as if making a sacrifice to the crocodiles in the moat. The second it went off fatigue cancelled out any energy to design strategies that might have helped. I wasn't particularly depressed by this because one day was pretty much like another and it became my new normal. Like a deep sea diver kicking up from the depths, I only surfaced when it was absolutely necessary. The blessing was that my young art students burst into my classroom with enough joy, and hugs, and enthusiasm to finally wake me up. And that "up" time, combined with God's help and learning to pace myself, resulted in success even when my brain fog made me forget those very successes! And, eventually things got much better.

How does one acquire this frustrating and disabling condition? There are many theories and more research is critically needed. One way is described by Dr's Oz and Rozen in their joint column, responding to this question: *"I'm 38, a wife and a working mom with three kids. My days are jammed. I'm worried about taxes; my boss wants me to take on more responsibility at work; the cellphone is always ringing. Sometimes I can't remember what I am supposed to be doing. It's scary to think I might have Alzheimer's disease already."*

The doctors replied: "Forgetfulness is a predictable result of a frantic daily schedule and a lack of downtime. It sounds like your brain fog is coming from two sources: The first source is the nagging stress of super-juggling—trying to fit all of your everyday responsibilities into an overcrowded schedule. The second source is information overload—what Alvin Toffler called 'infobesity' in his 1970 book *Future Shock*. And life's gotten a lot more info-obese since them. Today, it's well recognized that just as overeating damages your health, overconsuming information causes nagging, chronic stress. And all that stress can interfere with neural connections in your brain. In fact, studies have shown that multitasking makes each task take longer and causes more errors. The brain fog is real; fortunately, so is your ability to stop the problem. You've got to know your limitations."[3]

Chronic stress and sleep deprivation are very common causes of brain fog, but some medical conditions are also associated with this condition. For example, patients with fibromyalgia had ten times more loss of gray matter in the brain than people who are aging normally.[4] Other culprits that can cause brain fog include: thyroid disease, hepatitis C, candida, Lyme disease, tapeworms, and chronic fatigue syndrome. In addition, nutritional deficiencies (for instance an inadequate supply of protein, omega fats, vitamins, or minerals) can cause brain fog.

A toxic buildup of chemicals like copper or mercury is another cause and is becoming more prevalent as our environment becomes more polluted. Another contributor can be your medications. A significant number of over the counter and prescription medications, especially when combined, can cause brain fog for some people.

Depression is often linked to this condition, and it is a very common element of grief. C.S. Lewis described it this way in his classic, *A Grief Observed*: "At other times it feels like being mildly drunk, or concussed. There is a sort of invisible blanket between the world and me. I find it hard to take in what anyone says."[5]

> **SHARPER BRAIN TIPS**
>
> - Exercise first thing in the morning to reboot your brain.
> - Get enough sleep; brain fog can be caused by sleep deprivation.
> - Feed your brain cells a well-balanced, nutrient-rich diet.
> - With your doctor's help, analyze how your prescriptions and over-the-counter medications could be contributing to your brain fog.
> - At least one day a week, abandon your electronics and get out into nature to re-charge your spirit and refresh your mind.
> - Focus your mind through prayer and meditation. If you are a person of faith, seek to practice what the apostle Paul wrote to his disciple, Timothy, "But you should keep a clear mind in every situation . . ." (2 Timothy 4:5, NLT).
> - Limit multi-tasking; fog rolls in when you try to focus on more than one thing at a time.

41

Toxic Shocks

Our greatest joy-and our greatest pain comes in our relationships with others. — *Stephen R. Covey*[1]

IN A PERFECT WORLD, ALL OF OUR RELATIONSHIPS WOULD BE healthy, positive, and balance to our lives. Unfortunately, we don't live in a perfect world and not all of our relationships could be described as healthy. Some can more accurately be described as *toxic*.

Bad, sure, you muse. *Codependent, maybe. Intolerable would be getting closer. But toxic—as in poisonous?*

You're the only one who can determine this, so ask yourself:

- When you're with someone, do you feel energized or drained? Toxic people will squeeze the life out of you and leave you drained.
- After you spend time with him/her, do you usually feel better or worse about yourself? Toxic people are quick to criticize and thrive on pointing out your inadequacies and flaws. They feel better about themselves when they tear other people down.

- Is there fairly equal give and take in the relationship? There are givers and there are takers. Toxic people are takers.
- Do you feel calm and content with this person, or is the relationship characterized by constant drama? Toxic people thrive on drama and will create it where it doesn't exist.
- Can you be yourself around this person, or do you feel you need to change to make him/her happy?
- Is this person able to turn any conversation into a word war?
- Could this person have an argument with a sign post?[2]

Stressful relationships can lead to physical health issues in the long-term, in children as well as adults. Research on stress in children "shows that healthy development can be derailed by excessive or prolonged activation of stress response systems in the body (especially the brain), with damaging effects on learning, behavior, and health across the lifespan."[3]

When you feel threatened, your body responds by increasing heart rate, blood pressure, and stress hormones, such as cortisol. When the threat has passed, these stress responses return to normal. If the threat is long-lasting, this can lead to damaged, weakened systems and brain structure.

Toxic emotions can negatively affect your physical and emotional well-being, as well as your long-term brain health. Old memories or early trauma are locked into your brain. "Toxic emotions of fear, sorrow, anger, etc. dredge up stories from your childhood or past relationships. These old stories are superimposed onto the current memory and relationship and that specific neural network is reinforced in your brain."[4]

So, how can you protect your health, especially your brain health, from toxic relationships? Research shows that these kinds of relationships are best consigned to history. The stress from toxic relationships that aren't terminated can cause inflammation, which in turn can lead to all sorts of health issues, including heart disease, high blood pressure, and cancer.[5]

It's important to focus on positive emotions (well-being, happiness, trust, compassion, etc.) that can help you develop positive neural connections, and this will help you develop the healthy relationships you want. Research shows that a focus on positive emotions can help change the structure of your brain.[6]

Wanda's early relationships were negative and traumatic. Even though she has had a successful career as an adult, the results of her past trauma greatly influenced her current emotions and relationships. Her early trauma manifested itself in an eating disorder, depression, phobias, and suicidal tendencies as an adult. As a result of obtaining effective treatment, she found that she was finally able to deal with past emotions in a positive way. Today Wanda is speaking and writing on her experience of finding healing for her damaged emotions.

Toxic relationships are characterized by insecurity, abuse of power and control, demandingness, selfishness, criticism, negativity, distrust, drama, and other negative behaviors and emotions.

Healthy relationships are characterized by compassion, security, safety, mutual loving/caring, respectfulness, and so on. They leave you feeling happy and energized instead of feeling depressed and depleted.

SHARPER BRAIN TIPS

- Recognize when you are in a toxic relationship.
- Believe that you deserve to be treated with love and respect. Seek professional help if you have negative thoughts and beliefs about yourself that you can't shake.
- Confront toxic behavior if it is occurring in a setting that is safe for you. Use "I" statements such as, "I feel that you criticize everything I do. When you do that, I feel devalued."
- If nothing you do or say changes the behavior, establish boundaries with the person to protect yourself, emotionally and physically (if necessary). This may involve a temporary, or even a permanent, separation from the individual or individuals.

42

Unbind Your Mind

Habit, if not resisted, soon becomes necessity.
– St. Augustine[1]

MOST OF US ARE WELL AWARE OF THE DANGERS OF ADDICtion to drugs or alcohol, as these have become rampant since the drug culture began in the 1960s and much has been researched and written about them. Although some may question whether an addiction is a "disease" or the sad result of a series of wrong choices, modern brain imaging shows that addicts' brains experience changes similar to those seen in people with brain-related diseases such as Parkinson's, Alzheimer's, or mental illness.[2]

According to Joseph Frascella, PhD, director of the division of clinical neuroscience at the National Institute on Drug Abuse, "Addictions are repetitive behaviors in the face of negative consequences, the desire to continue doing something you know is bad for you."[3]

We can become addicted, dependent, or compulsively obsessed with any activity, substance, object, or behavior that gives us pleasure. Addictions occur when a behavior is repeated to the point that it disrupts the normal balance of brain circuits that control rewards, memory, and cognition, leading to compulsive and uncontrolled behavior. In other words, we become hooked not so much on the activity, but on the feelings produced by the chemicals in our brains.[4]

With the use of sophisticated technology, scientists can see what goes wrong in the brain of an addict—which neurotransmitters are out of balance and what regions of the brain are affected. They are developing a more detailed understanding of how deeply and completely addiction can affect the brain. Researchers are learning not only the short-term effects on the brain, but also the long-term effects in areas such as learning. Dopamine appears to be the *key chemical* in developing and maintaining addictions.[5]

Some of the common characteristics among addictive behaviors include: obsession with an object, activity, or substance; seeking out or engaging in the behavior even though it causes harm; compulsively engaging in the behavior; loss of control over the behavior (drinking too much, buying eight new pairs of shoes, eating a whole box of cookies, etc.); doing the behavior in secret and away from others; denial of the behavior or the extent of the behavior; and, withdrawal symptoms upon cessation of the activity.[6]

Addiction research has focused mainly on substance abuse, but increased technology and the knowledge of brain chemicals and how compulsive behaviors affect the brain have led researchers over the past few years to also target research on the following:

> **Internet Addiction**—Those addicted to the Internet have been known to flunk out of school, repeatedly lose jobs, lose contact with friends and family, and spend hours at the computer without eating or sleeping.[7]

Sexual and Pornography Addiction—An estimated sixteen million people have a compulsive sexual disorder; most are men. These addicts have become dependent on neurochemical changes in the brain during sex and are consumed by sexual thoughts. "The neurochemical pro-cess that happens in the brain when viewing pornography provides a high equal to that of crack cocaine."[9]

Shopping Addiction—Shopping can cause a "high" from the dopamine in the brain that switches on. The person feels good and the behavior is thus reinforced. Just as alcoholics hide their bottles, or pornography is done in secret on the Internet, "shopaholics" hide their purchases. The consequences of too much shopping are obvious; many have experienced financial ruin as a result.[10]

Gambling Addiction—Gambling addicts tend to be males from middle to upper-middle class backgrounds, often with a family history of alcoholism, depression, or compulsive gambling. From time to time they may win, but inevitably they start to lose. During this losing cycle they deplete their cash reserves and will often then borrow from others to cover their bets. This may eventually lead to taking illegal loans or theft to cover debts. Alienation from family and friends, job loss, physical ailments, and even suicide are often the result.[11]

Remember: *Anyone* can have an addiction. It's best not to judge others or to think yourself immune. Followers of Jesus are to emulate him as we run the race of life: "So we must get rid of everything that slows us down, especially the sin that just won't let go. And we must be determined to run the race that is ahead of us. We must keep our eyes on Jesus, who leads us and makes our faith complete" (Hebrews 12: 1-2, CEV).

SHARPER BRAIN TIPS

- Ask: Do I need more of any activity or substance than I did in the past in order to feel satisfied?
- Evaluate: When I can't or don't engage in the activity or use the substance, do I experience "withdrawal" symptoms such as craving, or depression?
- Analyze: Do I use more of the substance or engage in more of the activity than I intend?
- Assess: Do I long to cut down or control the activity or use of the substance, but find that I cannot?
- Audit: Do I expend significant energy, time, or money in order to obtain the substance or to engage in the activity?
- Assess: Have I given up social, occupational, or recreational activities due to this condition?
- Determine: Am I not able to give up the action or substance even though I know it is harming me physically, emotionally, relationally, or spiritually?
- Admit: Have I ever lied to anyone about my misuse of the substance or the extent of the behavior?
- Decide: If something is controlling you; if so, seek help.

43

This is Your Brain on Canvas

Only when he no longer knows what he is doing does the painter do good things." – *Edgar Degas*

It seems obvious that artistic painting is not like doing math or working at puzzles. One reason that painting is so different is that it is grounded in a different region of the brain. There is a distinction between our "left brain" and our "right brain." The left and right hemispheres of the cerebral cortex each have their own manner of perceiving information and processing it. The right brain is responsible for much of your intuition, spatial perception, and the capability to multitask. The left brain handles and processes language, logic, and cognition of details. But the left brain-right brain dichotomy is by no means ironclad, and varies from one individual to another. For example, while the left brain is referred to as the "language center" of the brain, this is only true for 93 percent of us.[1] And, for many tasks that people accomplish every day, the left and right side of the brain must cooperate efficiently to arrive at a correct answer or to decide on a proper course of action.[2]

Studies on right brain health are difficult to find. This may be because right brain functions are harder to measure (e.g., imagination and how well someone perceives spatial orientation, or intuits emotions), and science is grounded in measuring things. It is also true that medical science must follow grant funding.

The reality is that our Western culture is much more interested in left brain health and performance than in that of the right brain. In other words, math and engineering are valued over creativity, art, and music. Education reform is centered on the "3Rs" (reading, writing, and arithmetic, which are largely left brain activities) and art is relegated to the proverbial back seat.

Lance is a pastor. He is a bit "tightly strung" and he knows this. Lance decided to take up painting as a form of therapy. He had always wanted to learn to paint, so he thought, *Why not give it a try?* To avoid the stress of taking classes, he decided to take up paint-by-number painting. He had a lot of stress, so he did a lot of painting.

After the walls in his house were covered with his artwork, the completed canvasses began to fill up his attic. Along the way, he developed some painting skills. He developed comfort with the brush. He learned how perspective was created on the canvas. He learned use of color. He learned what it was about a painting that pleased him.

 One day, Lance realized that he had changed. He wanted to choose his own subject matter and began painting on blank canvases. His works are now more than therapeutic; they are expressions of his inner self. His paintings give him pleasure and his occasional art shows are crowd pleasers. For Lance, painting started as left brain activity of following instructions and working within defined boundaries, moving sequentially from one pre-drawn shape to another.

Eventually, he integrated a strong right brain collaboration that was free of boundaries and instructions. His right brain imagined the whole, even while his left brain focused on the individual parts. Lance became an artist, painting what he wanted and how he wanted and doing it very well.

Right brain health is more than just the ability to appreciate or create art. In a study of patients with injured frontal lobes (part of the cerebral cortex), the patients with left lobe injuries were compared to patients having right lobe injuries. A test was administered, known as a rule-switching test, which is designed to cause people to make mistakes. Those with left frontal lobe injuries corrected 68 percent of their errors, while those with right lobe injuries corrected only 30 percent.[3] How the left and right brain perceive and interpret information is very different, and what the right brain contributes can be very important to everyday life.

Our post-industrial culture rewards left brain thinking, and for the most part, we are products of our culture. But consider the old expression "remember to stop and smell the roses." This is a call to make choices that are outside of our default patterns of living. Smelling the roses would first require the right brain to identify the rose, while the left brain would be trying to ruin the moment by cataloging the number of petals, the height of the pistil, the length of the sepals, and so forth.

Students of art are often fascinated by the journey artists take as they explore and express various techniques through their paintings. Artists' creations are windows into their inner selves and often tell their own unique life story.

In this sense, a picture really can be worth a thousand words, for as the famous preacher Henry Ward Beecher said, "Every artist dips his brush in his own soul, and paints his own nature into his pictures."[4]

SHARPER BRAIN TIPS

- Show and tell, just like you did in kindergarten. Show the art (can be someone else's art work); Tell why you like it. Hint: It can be your own finger painting!
- Post your kids' or grandkids' art prominently in your home. Remember, it's their soul on canvas.
- Visit an art gallery or museum and just sit before a masterpiece and savor the mastery.
- Imagine yourself as the artist expressing your alter ego as you create this wonder.
- Expand this experience by creating and writing out a fictitious conversation between the artist and a gifted and very inquisitive eight-year-old child watching the artist work.
- Thank the Maker for giving you a mind equipped to appreciate beauty of this kind.
- Stop and paint the roses; use words if you prefer.

44

Mind Your Head

Traumatic brain injury (TBI) is the leading cause of death and disability in Americans under the age of 45.[1]

THE FIRST TIME I (DAVE) SAW THE UBIQUITOUS UK WARNING sign, "Mind Your Head," it took me awhile to figure out I should duck. Maybe a sign with a duck on it might have worked better in my case.

Concussions occur when the brain is slammed into the inside of the skull, disrupting normal brain activity. They occur with regularity in football, despite recent advances in equipment and changes in the rules. NeurosurgeryToday.org estimates that among high school, college, and professional players the number of concussions is 300,000 annually.[2] Until relatively recently, this effect was more or less shrugged off as a part of a hard-hitting game that only "real men" should play until they couldn't take it anymore.

These days, things are changing. In early 2015, NFL linebacker Chris Borland, 24, retired because he valued his long-term brain health versus whatever short-term gains (measured in millions of dollars) the game might have to offer. "I just honestly want to do what's best for my health," the athlete explained. "From what I've researched and what I've experienced, I don't think it's worth the risk. I'm concerned that it you wait until you have symptoms, it's too late."

One of the formerly overlooked long-term effects of concussions, especially multiple concussions, is depression. For example, retired Super Bowl champion linebacker Ted Johnson experienced at least fifty concussions during his career, always returning to the game as quickly as possible. He retired, in part due to his depression, which was severe enough to keep him in bed, in the dark, for the better part of a year and a half.³

Dementia is another, much worse, possible long-term result of concussion. John Mackey, a football star receiver with the Baltimore Colts under Johnny Unitas, scored a seventy-five-yard touchdown in 1971 to help the Colts win Super Bowl V. Later, he was inducted into the Pro Football Hall of Fame. But today, the fame means little to either Mackey or his wife, who had to appeal to the NFL for help with the high cost of caring for John's severe dementia, symptoms of which began to exhibit themselves when Mackey, now sixty-eight, was in his early fifties. Mackey is one of about a hundred former players with severe dementia receiving help from what is called the "88 plan," in honor of John's jersey number. The fund provides up to $88,000 annually toward the cost of their care.

Dr. Robert Cantu, originator of the Cantu Concussion Guidelines, believes it will eventually be proven that the problems of Mackey and many of these players were caused by the hits they took on the field. When interviewed on the CBS show *60 Minutes*, Cantu said, "In reality, I suspect if their brains could be studied, and hopefully one day they will, that traumatic encephalopathy is what has caused this dementia." The NFL has recently mandated that a neurologist should determine when a player with a head injury can return to the game, though improvement in this arena is still needed, according to many ex-players who struggle with brain-injury related diseases and the prospects of a shorter lifespan than their non-football playing contemporaries.[4]

Yet 300,000 football-related concussions are just the tip of the iceberg of such injuries from all sports and recreation activities combined. There are between five and twelve times that number (1.6 to 3.8 million) of sports and recreation-related concussions annually in the United States, according to the CDC's National Center for Injury Prevention and Control.[5] In addition to football, these would include organized sports like soccer, baseball and softball, boxing, competitive cycling, hockey, horseback riding, racing motor vehicles, skiing, wrestling, martial arts, pole vaulting, rugby, and so on. Some of these require protective headgear, some do not. Sometimes even protective headgear does not protect the way one might expect.

Purely recreational forms of some of the above sports can result in brain trauma, with or without a helmet. Plus there are many other recreational activities that can produce a closed head brain injury, including bicycle riding, kayaking, skateboarding, snow skiing, snowboarding, surfboarding, sailboarding, rock climbing, rollerblading, and water skiing—any recreational activity in which your head can receive a hard enough knock or jolt for your brain to collide with the inside of your skull.

You don't even have to actually hit the outside of your head on anything. What matters is what happens between the outside of your brain and the inside of your skull. This was tragically illustrated by the death of actress Natasha Richardson, who died as a result of a fall while learning to ski in Montreal. She was not wearing a helmet, but reports stated that she did not actually strike her head on anything or show any sign of external injury. In fact, according to reports, she was awake, alert, communicating, and without any major symptoms.

I (Dave) can attest to the possibility of brain injury without an external impact, having experienced this once when I fell backward while loading a trailer. I didn't actually strike my head on the floor; but I did become very ill with the typical symptoms of concussion, including severe vomiting and diarrhea concurrently. I thought I had eaten some tainted food. But Ms. Richardson's death and my subsequent study into closed head injuries helped me realize what had really happened—and how fortunate I had been not to have left this life before we could complete a few more projects.

Despite the high incidence of head injuries from recreation and organized sports, the top three leading causes of head injuries in America are: auto accidents (passengers or pedestrians); bicycle and motorcycle accidents; and falls (children and especially the elderly).[6] Designing (or redesigning) homes using the principles of Universal Design can help prevent such accidents in the home.[7]

SHARPER BRAIN TIPS

- Wear that helmet, even if it seems uncool. Wear it EVERY time you do anything that could involve head injury: biking, skiing, snowboarding, skateboarding, rock climbing, motorcycling, horseback riding, and so forth.
- Just do it!
- Click that seat belt, even if you think you'll never need it.
- Strap kids in whenever an accident might cause them to hit their heads—from the car to the grocery cart.
- Mind your windows (at home and on the road), so young children cannot crawl through or fall through.
- Always remember that your brain is far more sensitive to trauma than you can possibly imagine ... and that in less time than it will take you to finish this sentence, you could experience closed head trauma that would leave you seriously injured.
- Mind your head, but when you duck, don't quack, or people may think you're "quacking up!"

45

Go Beltless

While some risk factors cannot be controlled—such as age, gender, and family history of stroke—there are many things people can do to reduce the possibility of stroke.[1]
– *John Gullotta, MD*
Chair of AMA's Public and
Preventative Health Committee

WE ALL WANT TO AVOID A STROKE. STROKE IS THE THIRD leading cause of death in the US, where over 143,579 die each year. It is also a leading cause of disability. The risk of having a stroke more than doubles each decade after age fifty-five.[2] A stroke can take your life, or just ravage your quality of life, since it can affect the way you talk, move, think, and how you eat and drink.[3] It can even affect emotions and the way you interact with those you love.

There is a "stroke belt" stretching across the Southeastern US The states involved are North Carolina, South Carolina, Georgia, Tennessee, Alabama, Mississippi, Arkansas, and Louisiana. Death rates there from stroke are a full 30-40 percent higher than in the rest of the country! A large study, called REGARDS, was begun about sixty years ago to help solve this dilemma. The investigation found that just residing in this beautiful part of the US does not in itself mean you will suffer a stroke, but that avoiding the cultural trap of unhealthy behaviors is crucial to stroke-proofing your brain if you live there. This trap includes an unhealthy diet and smoking, among other factors.

Dr. Stephen Page, one of the researchers, explains, "Smoking and that whole class of unhealthy behaviors may be more common in those areas (the Southeast). They are tobacco-producing states, and there are places in the South where smoking is more common, and high blood pressure and diabetes are higher. Diet and genetics can certainly play a role; genetics can interact with nutrition and change the way the genes are expressed. The 'Southern diet' of fried chicken, fried vegetables, fried potatoes, and fried everything else may contribute to the problem. Also lifestyle . . . exercise and healthy behaviors aren't as common," adds Dr. Page.[4] The bottom line of this study is that you can live in the stroke belt and not be any more likely to suffer a stroke if you make an effort to *live a healthy lifestyle.*

Prevention is the place to focus, so we need to learn about the risk factors and aggressively adhere to those factors that we *can* control.[5] Obviously, we can't control our gender, race, and family history. We can't control our age and present medical history. For example, if a person has had a heart attack or suffers from sleep apnea or atrial fibrillation (a condition in which the heart beats abnormally), they are at higher risk for stroke. Risk increases for everyone after age fifty-five. And recently women have edged ahead of men in number of strokes. The death rate for women from stroke is twice that of breast cancer.

For those who have any of these risk factors, it is even more imperative to alter those that *can be controlled*, such as not smoking, not using illicit drugs or excessive alcohol, consuming a healthy diet, getting enough physical exercise, and managing your weight.

Significant lifestyle changes can lower your stroke risk. Researchers studied four risk factors: high LDL (bad cholesterol), low HDL (good cholesterol), high triglycerides (blood fat), and high blood pressure. The study group was 4,731 people, all of whom had suffered a recent stroke or mini stroke. Those who reached the optimum level in all four categories were 65 percent less likely to have another stroke as compared to those who did not reach optimum levels. In general, the following levels are healthier:

- LDL to be lower than 70
- HDL to be higher than 50
- Triglycerides to be less than 150
- Blood pressure to be lower than 120/80.[6]

This study underlines how critical it is to partner with your doctor to get your cholesterol, blood fat, and blood pressure into a safe range and to keep it there. Knowing it is possible to dodge a stroke, even if you have already experienced one, provides a sense of hope and the determination to focus on a healthy lifestyle.

SHARPER BRAIN TIPS

- If you have high blood pressure, diabetes, or high cholesterol, learn how to manage them as well as possible. Do not deny or ignore these conditions.
- Study effective treatments, and practice them.
- Be aware that hormone replacement therapy (HRT) during menopause, or using birth control pills can increase the risk of a blood clot.
- Use of illicit drugs or alcohol in excess is linked to higher incidence of stroke for men and women.
- Obesity increases your risk of stroke, so it is critical to keep your weight within a healthy range.
- Control or reduce your stress. Chronic stress can increase your risk of stroke four-fold. "Type A" personality traits, including being overly competitive, quick-tempered, impatient, aggressive, or hostile by nature increase your risk of stroke two-fold.
- Choose a salad versus the "bloomin' onion; or the veggie medley versus the French fries. Every time.

… 46 …

Listen to Your Other Brain

*You have to master not only the art of listening to your head,
you must also master listening to your heart and to your gut.*
— Carly Fiorina[1]

SURPRISE! YOUR GUT HAS A BRAIN OF ITS OWN THAT CONTROLS many of your digestive functions. This amazing system is called the "Enteric Nervous System" (ENS) and is located all through the lining of the GI tract. It communicates with the brain via the spinal cord. The ENS "talks to" the brain in our head by way of a small number of command neurons, which allow it to both send and receive messages. In fact, there is a lively conversation going on most of the day as situations and experiences open up a chat line between our two brains.

The enteric nervous system is made up of a network of neurons, proteins, and chemicals which allow it not only to learn and remember, but also to produce our "gut feelings."[2] Have you ever had a "gut-wrenching" experience? Has an exchange of words with your boss made you feel nauseous? Have you pondered where the "butterflies" came from, or why people sometimes feel "choked with emotion"? Well here are some answers.

For the last few decades, gastroenterologists have been hard at work studying the intricate connections between the brain and the gut. The discoveries have amazed and convinced even the most skeptical and given birth to a fascinating new medical specialty called neuro-gastroenterology. One of the pioneers in this specialty, Dr. Douglas Drossman from the University of North Carolina, is considered the world authority in his field and has written over 400 books, articles, and abstracts. His research and treatment discoveries have given hope to countless patients suffering from disturbing stress-related brain-gut symptoms.

A recent publication on the patient's perspective highlights the critical importance of good communication and understanding between patients and the doctor as well as relatives and friends. The study confirms again the important role that decreasing stress and promoting good relationships play in improving quality of life.[3]

As a gastroenterologist, I (Jim) want to give you an insider's look at how these complex brain-gut interactions occur. The gut contains 100 million neurons and is connected to the brain by layers of specialized tissue. The vagus nerve is the stick shift and controls the volume of gastrointestinal activity. The gut is not only able to send signals to the brain but *receives* information and "requests" as well. It also acts as a sort of drug store for the body's needs. The enteric nervous system can dispense major neurotransmitters like dopamine and serotonin, as well as various endorphins (the body's natural tranquilizers) at a moment's notice. Also located throughout the GI tract are brain proteins, sensors, neuron nourishers, and immune system cells needed for various body functions.

With every meal we eat, the enteric nervous system springs into action to monitor the digestion process and determine how your chicken and mashed potatoes should be mixed and propelled. This is often the reason we are highly tuned in to our gut messages when negative information like pain and bloating make their way to our brain.

Our modern way of life is often filled with stressful situations. In fact 20 percent of our US population suffers from a stress-related brain-gut condition called Irritable Bowel Syndrome (IBS). Stress signals from the head's brain can alter nerve function and turn up the volume of serotonin circuits in the gut. This overstimulation can cause problems all through the GI tract such as trouble swallowing, heartburn, nausea, abdominal pain, altered bowel habits, or bloating. Jerry was a fifty-two-year-old worker for the United States Postal Service. He had been employed there for more than ten years, but a distressing set of physical symptoms was making it more and more difficult to perform his work. He had developed severe diarrhea along with abdominal cramping and was miserable at the prospect of having to stop numerous times while driving throughout the day to use a roadside restroom. Fearing he had cancer, Jerry finally agreed to see a physician. I (Jim) did a few tests and thankfully found no sign of tumors or inflammatory diseases. I sat down with Jerry and said, "Jerry, you are free of disease but have a classic case of Irritable Bowel Syndrome. This chronic brain-gut condition is what is causing your symptoms. Have you been under more stress lately?"

"Well," admitted Jerry, "Come to think about it, the symptoms started around the time the Post Office cut back on personnel and my work load skyrocketed. At the same time we also found my daughter needed surgery."

"It is not unusual that this extra stress was enough to trigger all your uncomfortable GI symptoms," I replied.

"Wow! I just am shocked to find out that there is a connection. I had no idea," he said.

"Let's get you started on medication and some dietary guidelines and see if we can get these symptoms quickly under control."

Jerry also agreed to see a counselor for some stress-reduction sessions. Within a month, Jerry's symptoms had started to improve and he was his happy-go-lucky self once again, no longer dreading each day of work.

> ### SHARPER BRAIN TIPS
>
> - Learn stress reduction techniques and don't hesitate to get counseling to help with difficult problems.
> - Exercise regularly as this reduces stress hormones and encourages healthy digestion and elimination.
> - If you smoke, here's another reason to stop. Smoking stimulates the GI tract. That can mean frequent diarrhea like Jerry experienced.
> - Limit or eliminate alcohol, since alcohol irritates the GI tract.
> - Surround yourself with positive people.
> - Remember, if your gut starts "complaining," pay attention.

47

Reinvent Yourself

Don't simply retire from something; have something to retire to.   – Harry Emerson Fosdick, pastor[1]

RETIREMENT IS SOMETHING YOU MAY BE LOOKING FORWARD to and planning for, especially if you have spent many years in the workforce on the same job or in the same profession. You may have dreams of traveling, spending time with family and friends, getting your house and yard in order, or playing a few more rounds of golf each year. If you have saved and planned for your retirement, you may be looking at early retirement before age 65.

Many of us remember our parents and grandparents and what it was like for them when they retired. Many were on a fixed income and didn't have discretionary money to do a lot of extra things. They spent the greater part of their days in front of the TV or sitting on the front porch. For most, there was no thought of working after retirement, so "retirement" became the time between work and when they died. Many of them also did not have access to leisure activities geared towards seniors that the elderly do today.

Times have changed and retirement is viewed differently by many. For those nearing retirement age, particularly Baby Boomers, retirement presents challenges. In a study done by AARP, of the seventy-six million Baby Boomers, the majority either can't or don't want to retire.[2] Leaving a job at 55, 60, or 65 and puttering around the house is becoming a thing of the past. Many people are delaying retirement or retiring differently. People live longer, have more energy, many are better off financially, and they want to stay active doing something they enjoy well into their golden years.[3]

I (Dave) see it this way. In the Bible, nobody retired, possibly because people didn't live long enough to qualify for social security. Moses kept going strong until he died. The same is true for every other saint or role model in the entire Scriptures. Applying this to myself in my mid-sixties, I ask: Why should I even want to "retire?" My life is full to the brim with creative activities that I hope will advance the cause of Christ. Whether it be writing books like this one, or helping previously unpublished authors get published, I can't see a time now or in the future when I would want to back away from anything I'm doing.

A study completed by the Shell Oil Company found that "People who retired early at age 55 had almost twice the risk of death compared to those who retired at age 60 or older or who continued working. The risk of early retirement was greater for men. Mortality improved with increasing age at retirement for people from both high and low socioeconomic groups. The health status of those who retired at 60, however, was similar to those who continued working at 60. Survival rates remained significantly greater for those who retired at 65 compared with those who retired at 55."[4]

Health factors may have contributed to early death of those who retired early, but mental health may have been a bigger factor. Working represents something to do, a connection with others, something with purpose and meaning, a place to belong. Work offers the opportunity to keep the brain stimulated and active, and helps stave off depression.

As you plan for retirement, look at what many people are doing and consider "reinventing" yourself. What does this look like? Kelly Carmichael Casey, a career counselor in Portland, Oregon, who works with Baby Boomers, said that, "The expectations are that most of us need to continue to earn money after the traditional retirement age. Working has to have meaning and it has to feel as though it makes an impact in a positive way in the world."[5]

Remember, a second career can be the best retirement, especially if you are doing something you love, something that keeps you physically active, mentally stimulated, socially connected, and spiritually rejuvenated.

SHARPER BRAIN TIPS

- Start planning your next "career" while you are still in your pre-retirement years.
- Volunteer. It's a wonderful way to keep yourself active, keep your mind stimulated, to feel that you are doing something with meaning and purpose and giving back.
- Make a list of things you want to do, things you can do, the money you will need to earn, and what the ideal retirement would look like to you.
- Mentor someone in your area of expertise. Let them build on the foundation that your own experience and wisdom have created. Your connection with the past can be their connection with the future.
- Take a weekend away in a place conducive to reflection and ask yourself these questions: 1. If I knew I had ten years to live, what would I really want to do during that time? 2. What might I do that would fulfill my purpose—my reason for being here?
- Find a way to do what you've always wanted to do, especially if you've always been kept from what you wanted to do by what you had to do.

48

Play with Half a Glass

Every waking moment we talk to ourselves about the things we experience. Our self-talk, the thoughts we communicate to ourselves, in turn control the way we feel and act.
— John Lembo[1]

WE ALL HAVE DAYS WHEN WE ARE DOWN. SOMETIMES IT'S hard to maintain a positive outlook when our job is demanding, the kids are sick, the dishwasher breaks down after a big meal, there are bills to pay and very little money, and on and on. It's easy to have a glass-half-empty attitude when that's how the glass looks. In reality, however, this glass-half-empty outlook is not good for your health—physically, mentally, socially, or spiritually.

"Keeping a positive outlook on life may be one of the most important things we can do to keep our brains healthy and ready for learning. How we view ourselves, how we perceive the world around us, and how we interact with others can have profound effects on our overall well-being and on our brains."[2]

Having a positive attitude, therefore, is important to you no matter what your current age or present situation. But, how do you manage this—on good days and bad days? How do you develop a glass-half-full outlook on life? It all goes back to your brain and reprogramming your thinking. Where do our negative and positive thoughts come from? They are based on our beliefs and are formed early in life. They are influenced by the beliefs we have about ourselves and those that others have about us. Beliefs, then, influence our thoughts, which influence our self-talk, which ultimately influences our attitudes and behaviors.

We need to examine our inner messages and our beliefs—that is, what we think and believe about ourselves and the world around us. It is important to examine our feelings about particular thoughts and to decide if those thoughts are *true* or *untrue*. The more true and real a thought is and the better you feel about it, the more you can make those thoughts occur with greater frequency.

Sharon grew up in an abusive home. She was an unwanted child who was frequently told she was useless and would never amount to anything. She believed this throughout her childhood and into her adult life *even after* she got her master's degree in education and became a very successful drama teacher, raised three very well adjusted and successful sons, and had a happy marriage. It was difficult for Sharon to believe that she was successful and worthwhile because of the messages she heard as a child. Her self-talk and behavior was often degrading to herself. It was only after several years of therapy that she learned how to stop those negative thoughts and to replace them with positive ones about herself. She has become a much happier, more positive person who can celebrate her successes because she knows she has earned them.

Negative thinking and self-talk often takes the form of black and white thinking; disqualifying the positive and focusing on the negative; magnifying your mistakes; feeling you should, ought to, or must; labeling yourself a loser when you make a mistake; filtering everything that happens through a negative filter; assuming negative emotions reflect the way things really are; and personalizing every event as though you are the cause of it. These are also known as "cognitive distortions" or distorted thought patterns.

It is also important that you don't undermine positive thinking with such ideas as, "I never do anything right," or "I am so stupid." Replace these phrases with more positive ones. "Sometimes I do stupid things, but I'm basically a smart person."

Studies show that positive thinking and self-talk help you to sustain a healthy immune system, help you to live longer, help you to be healthier in general, help you to age more gracefully, protect your heart, and reduce stress.[3]

A really good choice is to let your outlook be guided by this Scripture: "There are some great things to think about, even though the world around us is so evil. Things that are true and good, lovely and honest, just and pure—these are the kind of thoughts that deserve your focus. Dwelling on these thoughts will produce mental and spiritual health and overall well-being in your life."[4]

SHARPER BRAIN TIPS

Martin Seligman, PhD, the "father of positive psychology," and author of *Learned Optimism*, suggests the following mnemonic device for adjusting your outlook, here summarized:

- Name the ADVERSITY, or problem.
- List your BELIEFS. These are your initial reactions to the problem.
- Identify the CONSEQUENCES of your beliefs.
- Formulate a DISPUTATION of your beliefs. Pessimistic reactions are often overreactions, so start by correcting distorted thoughts.
- Describe how ENERGIZED and EMPOWERED you feel now.[5]

49

Scrabble® Your Brain

Ninety-five percent of this game is half mental.
– Yogi Berra, baseball legend[1]

OF COURSE YOGI BERRA WAS TALKING ABOUT BASEBALL, but did you know that playing games—board games, word games, card games, crossword puzzles, and computer games—is also good for your cognitive functions? So if you want to increase your mental powers and help ward off dementia and Alzheimer's, consider dusting off your chessboard, checkerboard, dominos, or Scrabble® game and going a few rounds with your family and friends.

Having a sharp mind and a strong memory depend on the "vitality of your brain's network of interconnecting neurons, and especially on junctions between these neurons called synapses. Since many of the brain changes that accompany aging and mental disorders are associated with deterioration or loss of synapses, learning ways to strengthen and protect these important connections may help you delay or avoid cognitive decline."[2]

Research has shown that a lack of stimulation is associated with a reduced number of synaptic connections in the brain.

One study suggests that seniors who enjoy a variety of intellectually challenging activities, such as playing games and solving puzzles, have a lower risk of developing dementia.[2] The secret is to vary your mental activities and not let them become rote or routine. In other words, if you are a crossword puzzle whiz and can do them while you sleep, you might want to add something else to your repertoire, such as word or number games, to keep yourself mentally challenged and learning something new. Anything that relies on logic, word skills, math, and so on will help improve your brain's speed and memory. There are hundreds of online games, ranging from solitaire and other card games, to puzzle and word games, which can keep you mentally stimulated and challenged as you perfect your skills.

Bill and Mona both had challenging careers, so when they decided to move into a retirement community they wanted to stay sharp mentally as well as physically. Mona described their strategy. "In addition to playing tennis several times a week," she said, "Bill and I seized the opportunities all around us to stay challenged mentally. There are games and puzzles everywhere! As we wait for the elevator, we fit a few pieces into the 'puzzle in progress' located in each residence. There are Wii tournaments in our retirement residence, and we all try our hand at sports or even try learning to play an instrument. Opportunities for card and computer games abound. Recently something new has been started here at Shell Point Retirement Community (Ft. Myers, Florida) that has everyone talking. It is a five-week-long seminar on the brain! It is amazing how popular the class is. One friend went to the first class and said they could not wait 'til the second. It is so exciting and popular they hope to introduce it throughout the entire state. They will even train you to be a teacher!

"A book called *The Memory Bible*, by Gary Small, was recommended and Bill and I are going to the bookstore to get it this week. The teachers suggest that all of us should get a memory test, which is covered by Medicare. After all, we go for all kinds of physical tests, so why not include memory? I think it is a good idea, so I am going to encourage Bill to go and we can take it together. In addition to all this, our retirement community is going to introduce their plans for 'Big Brain Academy,' based on Nintendo software. One of our friends already started. He said his driving improved a great deal after doing the program regularly. He also was thrilled to find his focus and concentration improving. Another friend said their ability to do Sudoku improved. I am definitely going to volunteer to help out!"

How about video games? They're not just for kids anymore. Scientists are beginning to recognize the cognitive benefits of playing video games: creativity, pattern recognition, system thinking, decision-making, perception, and even patience. "Video games change your brain," said University of Wisconsin psychologist C. Shawn Green, who studies how electronic games affect abilities. So does learning to read, playing the piano, or navigating the streets of London, which have all been shown to change the brain's physical structure. The powerful combination of concentration and rewarding surges of neurotransmitters like dopamine strengthen neural circuits in much the same way that exercise builds muscles. But "games definitely hit the reward system in a way that not all activities do," he said.[4]

If you "Google" brain training and fitness web sites, you will find several that have a variety of games and activities. Lumosity.com and HAPPYNeuron.com offer a variety of challenging games and activities for a small monthly fee. Many sites are free. Of course games can be addicting just as anything else can be, but the goal here is to challenge your brain, to improve short-term memory and concentration, and to have fun in the process.

Many "seniors" have discovered the benefit of solving riddles, doing word puzzles, and mental math—"brain jogging," that helps them to think critically and stay sharp. These activities can also be a good way to meet others and to work as a team. So have fun online, or look for a brain workshop near you!

SHARPER BRAIN TIPS

- Step up your game. While it can feel relaxing to grab the same word search puzzle book when you need a break, push yourself to tackle more challenging exercises like brain teasers, Sudoku, or even Bridge. Your brain is forming new connections while it is puzzling over more difficult problems.

- Cross-train your brain. Athletes know how important it is to build their bodies by exercising different muscle groups. The same is true for the brain. When choosing brain games, look for activities that challenge your memory and attention skills. Next, add in other games that stimulate your verbal fluency, problem-solving skills, and creativity.

- Set the egg timer. Brain games are an important part of building a brain-healthy lifestyle. Block twenty minutes each day to get serious about brain games. Early morning is a great time to play games.

- Keep it social. Enjoy socializing while you play Canasta or Yahtzee®. Studies show that socializing enhances verbal abilities as we age and plays an important role in maintaining our brain's performance.

- Grab your favorite electronic device. Look for online options that tell you what skills you are working and allow you track your performance over time. Remember that short games with simple graphics can be just as beneficial as more complicated games with longer learning curves.

- Try a double scoop. If you are short on time, or looking for a new challenge, why not blend physical exercise with brain games. The children in your life will show you how. There are a number of amazing products out there that blend physical movement with problem-solving tasks. Some of the best options come from Wii-Fit and XBOX-360.[5]

50

Welcome to Club Med

Medicines can be your best friend or worst foe. – Unknown

THERE IS NO DOUBT THAT MEDICATION CAN BE A GREAT ALLY in our quest to live a high-quality life. Medicines have usually been associated with cure or symptom relief and taken with little thought about adverse effects. But the truth is that as more and more exotic drugs are discovered every year and made available in prescription form or over-the-counter (OTC), some are having unwelcome and even dangerous side effects. Add to that the growing search for herbals to enhance our quest for good health and we have a potential lurking menace.

Most of us can avoid a dangerous outcome just by discussing all the medicines and herbals we are consuming with our health care provider who can then, with his/her expertise and advanced medication software, help us guard against bad outcomes. Pharmacists are also taking up the challenge by putting time and energy into providing educational materials designed to alert us to potential problems with any new medicine. However as gerontologists search for ways to avoid the traps of aging, they are becoming concerned about the fact that 50 percent of the adult population use medicines every day that could have negative effects on their aging brains.

Some older folks ingest five or more prescriptions daily, and people who love them worry about a possible meltdown or megadose if someday the pill box that holds their daily doses gets lost or spills all over the floor. The problem is called "polypharmacy," and it is a contributor to the deaths of 100,000 older adults annually, according to one article.[1] The problem also affects younger people who may take a variety of OTC supplements in addition to their prescriptions, or add some other substance into the brain-pickling cocktail.

Laura was determined to do all she could to stay sharp mentally and had heard so many testimonials about herbal medicines that she decided to try one of the popular ones. Unfortunately she did not check with her doctor, and she took an herbal with blood thinning properties along with her daily Coumadin. She soon developed slight oozing into her brain that required a hospital admission to control. Laura recovered, but now much wiser, only takes herbal medicines with her physician's knowledge.

A study at the University of Illinois determined that commonly used medications may produce cognitive impairment in older adults. Some medications routinely used to treat medical conditions associated with aging (such as allergies, hypertension, asthma, and cardiovascular disease) appear to affect the brain in negative ways. The drugs studied included very popular OTC medicines like antihistamines, some antidepressants, sleep aids, itching remedies, and digestive and urinary tract aids.[2]

Sam developed severe allergies upon moving to a lush area of the country where beautiful trees and flowers flourished, but caused him increasingly disturbing symptoms. He suffered from stuffy nose, headaches, and sinus pressure and turned to his local drugstore for relief. He was elated when the OTC medicine relieved his symptoms. It wasn't long, however, before Sam began noticing he was having problems concentrating at work and his keen memory for names seemed to be diminishing. Concerned about his job performance, he went to his physician and learned that his "allergy medicine" was the culprit. A change to a different remedy restored his memory and concentration, and a grateful Sam learned to be cautious about treating symptoms on his own.

I (Jim) am often concerned about elderly patients who are taking prescription medications for anxiety long-term, because the medication can sometimes build up in the body, making it necessary to lower the dose to continue a safe range. Some common side effects in addition to memory and concentration problems are dry mouth, confusion, blurry vision, constipation, dizziness, and changes in bladder control. Some OTC medicines like antihistamines can also impair driving. Many herbals are a great benefit, but you must be certain they are not reacting with another medicine or herbal you may be taking. Patients with chronic pain often benefit from treatment in a pain clinic so that medication can be safely prescribed and monitored.

The Seattle Times reported that "more die from drugs than traffic accidents. Drug overdoses now outpace traffic accidents as the leading cause of injury-related death in 16 states, including Washington, as use of prescription painkillers continues to rise."[3] In addition, the recent concern over the under-treatment of debilitating effects of chronic pain has ushered in an increase in the use of opioids such as OxyContin. According to the University of Washington these opioids such as OxyContin, Vicodin, and Percocet are prescribed to one in five adults and one in ten adolescents annually. A study conducted by Group Health Cooperative concluded that the number of people taking opiates daily has risen from 2 to 4 percent. This means that one in twenty-five adults is now taking this class of drugs every day.[4]

Patients taking opioids are carefully cautioned about the potential dangers of the medications' effect on driving and are advised to avoid the potentially deadly combination of pain medication and alcohol. But way too many of them ignore those warnings and take to the road, putting themselves and others at unnecessary risk when they do.

> **SHARPER BRAIN TIPS**
>
> - Ensure that all prescribing persons are aware of every medication and OTC product the person in question is taking.
> - Read every insert that comes with prescriptions with a view toward possible side effects or interactions with the person's other medications and OTC products.
> - List any side effects you believe you have observed in the person in question.
> - Have all prescriptions filled at the same place; request information about interactions.
> - Whenever possible, transfer all prescribing to one physician, who can then track possible problems, while keeping the other doctors informed.
> - Carefully monitor every daily pill box in your home.

51

The Secret of Staying Focused

A well-orchestrated "executive brain" knows its priorities.
— Adam J. Cox, PhD[1]

THE MOST IMPORTANT FUNCTIONS THAT OUR BRAIN PERforms are the ones that make us who we are, wielding executive control and mediating our ability to focus in spite of life's distractions. The brain's CEO areas not only help us focus but also enable us to consciously study and retain information and behave appropriately as settings change. These areas of the brain are primarily located in the prefrontal cortex and are important because they are often tied to cognitive decline in aging. Our ability to memorize, plan, schedule, and juggle multiple tasks has its roots here. Recent studies are showing that these areas of the aging brain, with training, can end up reacting pretty much the same as in younger adults.

Research at the University of Illinois at Urbana-Champaign shows that brain training reignites key areas, boosting performance. Participants in this study were thirty-two men and women, ages fifty-five to eighty, and thirty-one younger adults. They were divided into control and experimental groups and run through a battery of brain testing. Before and after results showed significant improvement in the prefrontal cortex area in both the old and the young. Researchers commented that the old and young react in very much the same way with this type of training, thus countering aging factors.[2]

So we really are never too old to learn new skills.

In addition to brain training, researchers continue to report that aerobic exercise can prevent and possibly even reverse decline in these key areas of "executive control." The exercise must be strenuous enough to make a person slightly "breathless" and should be continued for at least thirty minutes (but should never be started without an okay from your physician). This type of exercise can not only improve the way the brain functions, but it also increases the volume of brain tissue. It has been shown that after only about six months of aerobic exercise people with age-related brain decline show evidence of their brain "plasticity" or capacity growing and developing.[3]

A crucial role of our brain's CEO is to trigger safe behavior and keep us from harm. This area of the brain seems to be more concerned about the consequences of our actions than how hard they are to produce. One theory is that our CEO is constantly monitoring itself so that appropriate actions or change of direction can take place. "Ability to realistically appraise our behavior at all times is especially important as we face dangerous or technically difficult situations. Executive functions are often invoked when it is necessary to override responses that may otherwise be automatically elicited by stimuli in the external environment."[4]

Anyone who has ever been on a diet is familiar with this struggle. You see a big piece of apple pie and you want it. Your CEO clicks in and tries to inhibit this automatic response! There can be a bit of a tug-of-war. One way researchers can test executive function control is by using flash cards that have the names of colors printed on them but in different ink colors.

For instance the word purple may be printed in green ink. This presents our CEO with a dilemma. If asked to say what you see, your automatic response would be to say the word, "purple." But you would have to override the automatic response when asked to look at the card and name the color in which the word is printed. Or how about when you move to a new neighborhood and find you have automatically driven home to the old house? Or, much more serious, you are driving and a text comes in from your best friend and you decide to focus on reading and answering it?

As you would expect, when attention is being diverted to texting, the brain's CEO is occupied and unable to detect dangerous but subtle changes. For instance, if we are paying close attention while at the wheel, we will notice that the light is about to change or there is a car approaching rapidly from the rear, or a car on the left is making slight movements toward our lane, or a small child is running toward the street.

Failure to detect hazards and respond quickly increases stopping time by three car lengths. This distance can make the difference between causing or avoiding an accident and between fatal and non-fatal consequences. Losing focus while driving also makes the driver unable to maintain consistent safe distance from other cars as well as staying in their own lane.

So, don't become part of a gruesome statistic, as did 19-year-old Daniel Schatz, who received or sent eleven texts while driving, the last of them just before he was killed when his pickup crashed into the back of a tractor trailer cab, creating a chain reaction involving two school buses. The buses were carrying nearly fifty students to an amusement park outing.

One bus-riding student was killed and thirty-eight others

were injured in the Missouri crash. When you're driving, or whatever you're doing, stay focused or things could turn out far different from what you had in mind.

SHARPER BRAIN TIPS

- Organize your thoughts before you start something. Make notes for your "CEO," if needed.
- Anticipate as realistically as possible the space and tools and time the task may require.
- Manage your time well by establishing priorities and sticking to them—this is especially important when you are using the Internet.
- Even when intently focused on a task, retain enough flexibility to adapt if the situation changes; for example, an "interruption" may actually help solve something you're working on.
- Try not to over-react to obstacles, since your emotions may hinder your progress toward a solution.
- Memorize the information you need to remember —but back up your brain by filing the information somewhere else, also.
- Remember: Singlemindedness is a character trait of those who accomplish much, like the apostle Paul, who said, ". . . one thing I do: forgetting what lies behind and reaching forward to what lies ahead, I press on toward the goal for the prize of the upward call of God in Christ Jesus" (Philippians 3:13-14, NASB).

52

In Spirit and in Truth

> *God is spirit, and his worshipers must worship in spirit and in truth.* — Jesus (John 4:24)

EVERYONE WORSHIPS SOMETHING. AND WHAT WE WORSHIP has a deep effect on our health, including the health of our minds. According to psychiatrist Timothy R. Jennings, the drive to worship is "an inherent part of our being . . . experienced by everyone, whether they admit it or not. It might be the Dallas Cowboys, money, power, a pop culture figure such as Madonna, the scientific method, or oneself. But everyone worships something."[1]

To this list we might add a variety of other things that people worship, including sex, fame, one's spouse or family, external beauty, automobiles, NASCAR cars and drivers, Indy cars and drivers, yachts, houses and properties, technologies, politicians and their ideologies, religious leaders and their ideologies, Hollywood personalities, TV, heroes (athletic and otherwise), rock music, classical music, psychedelic experiences, physical fitness, health, longevity, relics, saints, ancestors, hunting, fishing, surfing, rats, golden calves and sacred cows, even shoes . . . the list of things people are willing to consider sacred is as long as the number of people in the world is large.

An article I (Dave) received while creating this chapter included a conversation between the missionary doctor and the patient, who responded to the question, "What do you worship?" by pulling a little jade Buddha from her pocket. "This is what I worship," she replied.

In Athens, in the apostle Paul's day, there was an altar in the Areopagus to "an unknown god."[2] And the apostle used that innate belief—that there was something greater—to speak of Jesus and the gospel.

All human beings are religious to one degree or another, if by "religious" we mean that they exhibit a certain level of faithful devotion to an ultimate reality or deity. The Judeo-Christian tradition is clear on the reason for this, since both Old and New Testaments describe this innate human need to worship and the consequences of worshiping truth versus a lie.

For example, the Old Testament prophet Isaiah wrote: "Half of the wood he burns in the fire . . . From the rest he makes a god, his idol; he bows down to it and worships. He prays to it and says, 'Save me; you are my god.' They know nothing, they understand nothing; their eyes are plastered over so they cannot see, and their minds closed so they cannot understand. No one stops to think, no one has the knowledge or understanding to say, 'Half of it I used for fuel; I even baked bread over its coals, I roasted meat and I ate. Shall I make a detestable thing from what is left? Shall I bow down to a block of wood?' He feeds on ashes, a deluded heart misleads him; he cannot save himself, or say, 'Is not this thing in my right hand a lie?'" (Isa. 44:16–20).

The New Testament is equally clear: "For since the creation of the world God's invisible qualities—his eternal power and divine nature—have been clearly seen, being understood from what has been made, so that men are without excuse. For although they knew God, they neither glorified him as God nor gave thanks to him, but their thinking became futile and their foolish hearts were darkened. Although they claimed to be wise, they became fools and exchanged the glory of the immortal God for images made to look like mortal man and birds and animals and reptiles. . . . They exchanged the truth of God for a lie, and worshiped and served created things rather than the Creator—who is forever praised. Amen. . . . Furthermore, since they did not think it worthwhile to retain the knowledge of God, he gave them over to a depraved mind. . . ." (Rom. 1:20–28).

Since all humans in all ages have worshiped something, there is obviously an innate drive in this direction. If you accept the idea of a Creator God, then it seems logical to accept that the Creator made us this way. If you do not accept the concept of a Creator, or Intelligent Design, or whatever you wish to call it, then you simply cannot explain this drive, whether you appeal to Freud, Marx, Darwin, or anybody else.

The only way to solve this conundrum is to accept that God really is, and this truth will set you free. Of course, each individual is free to choose what he or she will worship. And we really mean it when we say that you're welcome to believe what you want to believe.

But if you want peace of mind, and health of mind, you'll survey all of history and all of religion, philosophy, and psychology, and any other discipline, and you'll see that in the end there was one person who was unique. He lived to show us what God is like. He died so we might be able to have life to the full. And he rose again from the dead to defeat our ultimate adversary, death, and to prove that through faith in him, all can be well (now) and will be well (forever) in body, soul, and mind.

SHARPER BRAIN TIPS

- Ask God to help you to strengthen your relationship with him.
- Read God's love letter, the Bible, thoughtfully and often.
- Consider writing a short letter back God relating to what you have read.
- Analyze how you are spending your time. Identify activities, including "religious" activities, that may be stealing time you might otherwise spend in worship.
- Be courageous enough to back out of some activities, if necessary.
- Open yourself to knowing God more intimately and to being known by him.

Keep in mind this key thought:
Enjoy God and love him forever!

Conclusion

If Your Brain Could Talk, It Would Say:

FEED ME

Your brain consumes 20 percent of the fuel you provide your body. So your question is what grade fuel are you going to feed it: Regular, Mid-Grade, or Premium? Or are you feeding Diesel fuel to a non-Diesel tank, making it sputter and malfunction? Your Maker designed your mind for high performance, and has recommended that to help it perform well, you should consume premium fuel, which comes from whole foods, including a wide variety of vegetables, fruits, berries, grains, seeds, and nuts. Protein from sources such as dairy products, eggs, fish, poultry, and other meats is best thought of as a "garnish," as Ben Franklin suggested. If you supplement, do so wisely. Base your decision-making not on stories from anyone, or claims made by supplement making companies, but from double-blind, placebo-controlled, randomized scientific investigations conducted by independent researchers and published in peer-reviewed journals.

Bottom line: Eat whole food that is as close to its natural state as possible; avoid food-like substances that come already prepared for your convenience.

WALK ME

Your brain came with a body that needs to move. With few exceptions, we choose day by day how much we will do that. Statistics show a lot of really bad trends in terms of physical exercise in America. You are the only person who can take yourself out of that box. If you really want a sharper brain, get moving, because physical exercise:

- Improves overall brain health, most likely as a result of increased blood flow.
- Lift your mood, and help combat depression, if you struggle with that.
- Increases the production of the specific growth factor (BDNF) that nourishes and supports brain cells.
- Enhances the production of neurons in the hippocampus, and also the number of cells produced to protect and support neurons.

Bottom line: Get off the couch; take your brain for a walk.

CHALLENGE ME

Your mind values something to do. The Religious Orders Study has found that participants who more frequently engaged in activities such as listening to the radio, reading newspapers, playing puzzle games, going to museums—i.e. staying actively engaged with their world—have a lower incidence of Alzheimer's disease.[1]

Brain training can also help, whether in person or online. Studies are showing long- and short-term benefits such as improvement of attention, memory, and processing speed.[2] Your main questions will be whether and how much you are willing to pay to enlist in one or more of the online brain training programs. Yes, some programs are free. But you get what you pay for, of course.

Bottom line: Work at it. Gain and pain are linked.

REST ME

In today's digitized, nonstop existence that is focused on productivity in a 24/7 global environment, it's tempting to believe that you can increase your output by taking your work with you everywhere you go—home, on vacation, to church, to bed, wherever you can get a high speed connection. Your mind, however, was not designed for this kind of life. A full night's sleep is a crucial pillar of health in general, and brain health in particular. Your brain does not turn off during this time . . . far from it. While you rest, your brain is consolidating and filing all the new information you just gave it. When it is deprived of this opportunity, your cognitive abilities suffer.

Bottom line: All work and no sleep will make you less efficient and less effective over time.

CHILL ME

Life is full of stress—some good, some potentially destructive. Even good stress can become dis-tress if you have no energy margin to deal with it. For example, the process of building a new home (good stress) often produces significant distress in the relationship of those building it. Relentless pressure produces cortisol, which damages cells in your hippocampus, and inhibits retrieval of information you've already stored. You can learn to manage your stress, by taking control of what you can control—for example, your attitude and your outlook. Stress-reduction techniques have been shown to be effective antidotes to stress. In the words of St. Augustine: "I pray thee, spare thyself at times: for it becomes a wise man sometimes to relax the high pressure of his attention to work."

Bottom line: It is possible to experience serenity even in the midst of stressful situations, and thus relax your body, mind, and spirit.

CENTER ME

Anxiety and depression are brain assassins. Their specific effects can be seen through MRI scanning—damage to the hippocampus, anterior cingulate, and prefrontal cortex. By contrast, having faith in a personal God can be the source of a peace that transcends human understanding: "Don't fret or worry. Instead of worrying, pray. Let petitions and praises shape your worries into prayers, letting God know your concerns. Before you know it, a sense of God's wholeness, everything coming together for good, will come and settle you down. It's wonderful what happens when Christ displaces worry at the center of your life" (Philippians 4:6-7, MSG).

Bottom line: Let Christ displace worry at the center of your life.

CONNECT ME

As some people age, they gradually withdraw and over time become increasingly isolated. Loneliness can creep in. Studies have shown that the brains of lonely people react differently from those with strong social networks. Why? No one really knows for sure. Perhaps when you're connected with a network of people who share common interests, you know that there is, in the words of one pioneer in the field of personal wholeness, Swiss physician Dr. Paul Tournier, "A Place For You." When there's a place for you, you are more likely to provide "a place" for others. You have their backs; they have yours. So whatever life brings your way, you don't have to face it alone. Knowing that you fit in, that your life makes a difference, gives a sense of purpose and life satisfaction that is one of the keys to psychological, sociological, and spiritual wholeness.

Bottom line: Nurture mutually supportive relationships.

And now . . . the rest of the story of love . . . and hope . . . and faith.

Perhaps you were wondering what happened to Dr. Walt Larimore's daughter, Kate, who faced some overwhelming challenges from her very first days of life. While some medical "experts" offered advice that assumed the worst, and were based on pessimism, the Larimores never gave up hope that "Love Works Miracles." The following is by Dr. Larimore, and from his perspective:

You can imagine my concern and frustration—I had no idea what was waiting. Had Barb decided to leave me? She sure had every justification. Was Kate hurt? Had she fallen?

When I arrived home, I found no ambulances in the driveway. I rushed in. There in the living room, I saw Barb and Kate sitting together. Barb was weeping. Kate was smiling.

"Barb, what's the matter? What's wrong?"

Barb just silently gestured to me to come over and sit by her. "Watch," she whispered. Kate giggled. "Let's show Daddy, Kate." Barb took her other hand and helped our physically disabled child stand. Kate was laughing and smiling from ear to ear.

Then I watched Kate take her first step. The child who they said would never walk, walked. And, I was the one who cried like a baby.

Kate did learn to walk. And, to talk. And, with many surgeries, to run. And, she's not stopped walking or talking since.

One day, while sitting on Barbara's lap, Kate looked up and asked, "Momma, does Jesus live in your heart?"

"Of course," her mom exclaimed.

Kate looked up and asked, "Can I listen for him?"

Surprised, and not really sure what to say, Barb whispered, "Of course."

As Kate bent her head over to Barb's chest, listening intently, her eyes widened like saucers. "Oh, momma," Kate spoke very softly. "I can hear him, I can hear him."

Her stunned mother exclaimed, "What do you hear, honey?"

Kate softly stated, "I hear him making coffee."

Well, it was on that same lap, at five years of age, that Kate—who we had been told would never walk or talk or run or think complex ideas, asked the Lord to come into her life. She asked him, who had fearfully and wonderfully made her, he who knew her before time, to come live in her heart, to be her Lord, to be her Savior.

Kate began a life of trusting her Creator and growing to intimately know him. He led her and her parents through eye surgery to straighten out a wandering eye. He grew and nurtured her mentally and spiritually—as he did her parents. He even gave her a brother to test her patience and ability to love others.

She went on to graduate in the top 10 percent of her high school class and was named as one of the nation's 100 Horatio Alger Scholars—for overcoming major obstacles on the path of becoming a successful role model. She went on to graduate from Samford University with a degree in English and Creative Writing. Afterwards, she served internships with an editor of Southern Living and in the speechwriting department at the White House for President Bush.

Her smile is radiant, her spirit sweet, her intellect sharp, and her humor dry. When I see her run or walk or laugh or talk, I am reminded of Isaiah 40:31 which says, ". . . those who hope in the Lord will renew their strength. They will soar on wings like eagles; they will run and not grow weary, they will walk and not faint."

I can imagine that when I see the Lord face to face, he will allow me to ask my "Why?" questions. He will, I believe, smile and ask me to look back upon my life, seeing it through his eyes. I will see how he interlaced my life with the lives of many others. I will see the lives he touched with each move he made. With glee and wonder, I will finally see just how it all fit together. I will, I suspect, turn back to him with amazement, tears of conviction and joy streaming from my eyes, lips quivering, and confess, "Lord, it was perfect!"

He will probably smile, and hug me, and wipe the tears from my eyes.

Then, I think he will lovingly say, "I know. Actually, I always knew it would be."[1]

About The Authors

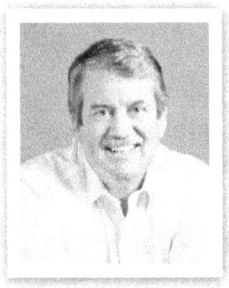

Dr. David B. Biebel is a minister, author, and editor. He holds a Doctor of Ministry degree in Personal Wholeness from Gordon-Conwell Theological Seminary. For nearly twenty years he served as editor for the Christian Medical & Dental Associations' flagship journal *Today's Christian Doctor*, before serving on the staff of Florida Hospital's Publishing division as Managing Editor until 2014. Dr. Biebel has authored or co-authored nineteen books, including three with the Dills. He founded Healthy Life Press in 2008 to help previously unpublished authors get their works to market. His hobbies include hunting (especially bowhunting for elk), fishing, camping, golfing, and cooking. He lives in Colorado.

James E. Dill, MD, was a board certified gastroenterologist with over forty years of practice experience. In Jim's latter years he enjoyed working as a locum tenens physician in a number of states including Hawaii. He co-authored three books including this one, *Your Mind at its Best*, and *The A to Z guide to Healthier Living*. While serving in Hawaii, he and his wife, Bobbie, made several medical trips to American Samoa to assist the physicians there in patient care. The Jim Dill Memorial Samoan Fund was established to help the Samoans

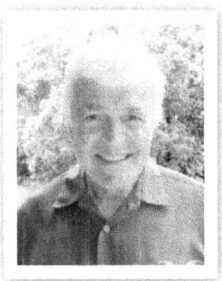

with access to care thru the Straub clinic and Hospital, 888 King St., Honolulu, HI 96813. His love for his family, friends, and patients enriched his world, and his dedication to whole person medicine will remain a legacy.

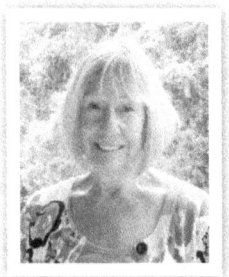

Bobbie Dill, RN, has served as a nurse in various specialties throughout her career with an emphasis on women's health, in which she holds a certification. She enjoyed many years of working alongside her husband in his medical practice, which was among one of the first to establish a truly wholistic medical emphasis, encompassing the medical, emotional, spiritual, and relational needs of patients. Bobbie enjoys writing and co-authored with her husband, Jim, nineteen journal articles and three books, including this one. She now resides in Virginia where she enjoys time with her family, including her three granddaughters, as well as serving in her church and community.

The authors' goal is to help people attain and maintain optimal health so they can love the Lord with their whole heart, soul, mind, and strength, and their neighbors as themselves.

Notes

Chapter 1: Stop Aiming and Shoot Already!
1. http://scan.oxfordjournals.org/content/early/2013/01/11/scan.nst004.abstract?sid=2583071a-85f7-4c51-b685-1956d84c88f7.
2. http://www.nytimes.com/2011/08/21/magazine/do-you-sufferfrom-decision-fatigue.html?pagewanted=all&_r=0.
3. Maria Szalavitz, "Making Choices: How Your Brain Decides" (*Time*: Sept. 4, 2012). http://healthland.time.com/2012/09/04/making-choices-how-your-brain-decides/#ixzz2Vkedh4vg.
4. http://www.gha.net.au/Uploadlibrary/3932160003-GriefCopingwithChallenges.pdf.
5. Jan Gläscher, Ralph Adolphs, et al. "Lesion mapping of cognitive control and value-based decision making in the prefrontal cortex." *Proceedings of the National Academy of Sciences of the United States of America* (Vol. 109, No. 36, Sept.4, 2012), 14681-14686. See: http://www.pnas.org/content/109/36/14681.full.pdf+html.
6. http://www.nature.com/tp/journal/v2/n7/abs/tp201259a.html.
7. Dr. Daniel Amen, *Healing the Hardware of the Soul* (New York: Free Press/Simon and Schuster, 2002), 150. To learn more about Dr. Amen's programs, visit: www.theamensolution.com.
8. http://99u.com/articles/7043/dont-overthink-it-5-tips-for-dailydecision-making.

Chapter 2: To Sleep Perchance to Dream
1. Shakespeare (Hamlet, Act 3, Scene 1).
2. *Time* magazine correspondent and neurosurgeon Dr. Sanjay Gupta, as quoted in: http://www.time.com/time/magazine/article/0,9171,1169907,00.html.
3. http://online.wsj.com/article/SB10001424127887323301104578257894191502654.html.
4. Noh and group, *Journal Clinical Neurology* (2012 more specific citation needed)
5. This quiz was created by the authors, based on a survey of ideas on this subject. It has not been tested scientifically.
6. http://www.ninds.nih.gov/disorders/brain_basics/understanding_sleep.htm#dynamic_activity.
7. http://www.journalsleep.org/ViewAbstract.aspx?pid=28123.
8. http://store.brightkey.net/nsf_ebiz/OnlineStore/ProductDetail.aspx?ProductId=29.

Chapter 3: Why'd I Come in Here?
1. "Scientists Show Hippocampus's Role in Long Term Memory," Science Daily, 2004, www.sciencedaily.com/releases/2004/05/040513010413.htm.
2. Simon Wootton and Terry Horne, Training Your Brain (Blacklick, OH: McGraw-Hill Companies, Inc., 2007), 79.
3. "Researchers Show How The Hippocampus Records Memory," http://www.news-medical.net/news/2009/03/12/46843.ASPX.

Chapter 4: Wow Your Brain
1. From the home page of "Space, Science and Spirituality." See: http://www.chdr.cah.ucf.edu/spaceandspirituality/about.php.

2. David Hochman, "The Key to Fulfillment," at: http://www.oprah.com/health/The-Science-of-Awe-and-Fulfillment#ixzz2Veljf6Kn.
3. Melanie Rudd, et al. "Awe Expands People's Perception of Time, Alters Decision Making, and Enhances Well-Being." Psychological Science (Volume 23, Number 10, 2012), 1130-1136. PDF available at: http://www.carlsonschool.umn.edu/assets/lib/assets/AssetLibrary/2012/Rudd_Vohs_Aaker_2012_psych%20science.pdf.
4. Ross, Jerry; Norberg, John. *Spacewalker: My Journey in Space and Faith as Nasa's Record-Setting Frequent Flyer* (W. Lafayette, IN: Purdue University Press, 2013), Kindle Edition. Kindle Locations 3502-3508.

Chapter 5: Is this a Senior Moment, or . . . ?
1. Jean Carper, *Your Miracle Brain* (New York: Harper Collins, 2000), 23.
2. Daniel J. DeNoon, "Mediterranean Diet Plus Exercise Lowers Alzheimer's Risk," http://www.webmd.com/alzheimers/news/20090811/mediterranean-diet-plus-exercise-cuts-alzheimers-risk?page=1.
3. Majid Fotuhi, *The Memory Cure: How to Protect Your Brain Against Memory Loss and Alzheimer's Disease* (New York: McGraw-Hill, 2004), 170-177.

Chapter 6: Bring Back the Slide Rule
1. Note: Nobody lost; everyone was treated fairly. If you scored 100 (no one ever did), then that was your "square root x 10" score. But if you got a 64, you ended up with an 80; a 49 became a 70.
2. Simon Wootton and Terry Horne, "The Heirarchy of Thinking Skills," *Training Your Brain*. (Blacklick, OH: McGraw Hill Co., 2007), 61.
3. Society Today. "Children are falling behind in math and science."
4. http://www.esrc.ac.uk/ESRCInfoCentre/about/CI/CP/the_edge/issue21/maths_science.aspx.

Chapter 7: Just Dance
1. L. Baker, S. Craft, C. W. Wilkinson, P. Green, S. R. Plymate, G.S. Watson, B. Cholerton, L. Smith, and L. Fisher, "Six months of controlled aerobic exercise reduces cortisol for women but not men with MCI," *Alzheimer's and Dementia* (vol. 5, no. 4, supplement 1, July 2009): 334.
2. Y.C. Peia, S.W. Choua, P.S. Linb, Y.C. Lina, T.H. Hsua, and A.M. Wonga, "Eye-hand Coordination of Elderly People Who Practice Tai Chi Chuan," *Journal of the Formosan Medical Association* (107, Issue 2, February 2008): 103-10.
3. Source: "How to cut your risk of memory loss," by David S. Martin, CNN, and found at: http://www.cnn.com/2011/11/09/health/keeping-brain-youngmemory.
4. "Learning, Arts, and the Brain," The Dana Consortium Report on Arts and Cognition, http://www.dana.org/uploadedFiles/News_and_Publications/Special_Publications/Learning,%20Arts%20and%20the%20Brain_ArtsAndCognition_Compl.pdf.

Chapter 8: Get Engaged
1. "Taking Control of Brain Health: Stay Socially Connected," AARP, http://www.aarp.org/health/healthyliving/brain_health/articles/brain_socially_connected.html.

2. Ibid.
3. Tom Valeo, "Good Friends are Good for You," WebMD, http://www.webmd.com/balance/good-life-health-well-being-9/friends-relationships?print=true.
4. Some suggestions regarding socialization and brain health were found at: http://www.fitbrains.com/lifestyle/socialization.php.

Chapter 9: Stop Killing Yourself Slowly

1. "Can Unhealthy Food Hijack Your Brain?" CBS News, http://cbsnews.com/stories/2009/04/20/health/main4958349.shtml.
2. "Saturated Fats Can Cause Alzheimer's Disease," http://news-reviews.org/uncategorized/saturated-fats-can-cuase-alzheimers-disease/.
3. Information on this subject can be found at: http://en.wikipedia.org/wiki/Neurotoxicity.
4. Larry McCleary, "The Goldilocks Principle," (September 13, 2007, http://www.drmccleary.com/2007/09/13/TheGoldilocksPrinciple.aspx.
5. http://www.webmd.com/brain/news/20100520/too-much-bellyfat-linked-to-dementia.
6. http://www.scientificamerican.com/article.cfm?id=your-liver-may-be-eating-your-brain.
7. McCleary, op cit.
8. This list is based on the WebMD article: http://www.webmd.com/diet/features/eat-smart-healthier-brain.
9. For a list, and a comparison, see: http://www.askdrsears.com/topics/feeding-eating/familynutrition/nuts/health-nuts-ranking-nuts.

Chapter 10: Play Furniture Roulette

1. Pick the Brain, "Does Your Brain Need an Oil Change?" February 13, 2008, http://www.pickthebrain.com/blog/brain-fitness/.
2. http://www.ncbi.nlm.nih.gov/pmc/articles/PMC164689/.
3. Riley, Barbara, "Your Brain—Use it or Risk Losing It as You Age," Ohio Department of Aging, March 2009, http://aging.ohio.gov/news/agingissues/ai_2009_3a.asp.
4. Cortright, Suzie, "Simple Feng Shui: Eight Quick Ways to Redecorate for Your Spirit." All-Home Décor, March 2004, http://www.all-homedecor.com/fengshui.htm.

Chapter 11: A Concert State of Mind

1. Daniel Amen. "Healing the Hardware of the Soul." *Christian Counseling Today* 12, no. 3 (2004): 19-24.
2. Ibid.
3. Andrew Newberg and Mark Robert Waldman, *How God Changes Your Brain* (New York: Ballantine Books, 2009), 18-19.
4. Ibid., 27.
5. Andrew Newberg, M. Pourdehnad, et al, "Cerebral blood flow during meditative prayer: preliminary findings and methodological issues," *Perceptual & Motor Skills* (97, no. 2; 2003): 625-30.
6. From John Michael Talbot, *Come to the Quiet: The Principles of Christian Meditation* (New York: Tarcher, 2002), 20-21.

Chapter 12: Stoke Your Belly Fire
1. Denise C. Park, Angela H. Gutchess, Michelle L. Meade, and Elizabeth A.L. Stine-Morrow, "Improving Cognitive Function in Older Adults: Nontraditional Approaches," *Journals of Gerontology*: SERIES B 62B (Special Issue I, 2007): 45–52.
2. K.M. Lang, D. Llewellyn, I. Lang, D. Weir, R. Wallace, M. Kabeto, and F. Huppert, "Cognitive Health Among Older Adults In The United States and in England," *BMC Geriatrics* (2009, 9): 23.
3. Lewis Lajos Incze. *Footprints on Destiny Lane* (Lisbon Falls, Maine: Beacon Press) 1982.
4. S.L. Willis, et al, "Long-term Effects of Cognitive Training on Everyday Functional Outcomes in Older Adults," *Journal of American Medical Association* (296:23): 2805-14.
5. John J. Ratey, MD, with Eric Hagerman, *Spark: The Revolutionary New Science of Exercise and the Brain* (New York: Little, Brown and Company, 2008), 242-243.

Chapter 13: How Do You Want Your Change?
1. This segment is based on our observation and personal experience with hundreds of doctors like Phillip, who rarely stop to ask the questions raised until some life crisis forces them to stop and rethink where they've been headed, and to change the habits of thought that have controlled that direction.

Chapter 14: A Funny Thing Happened on the Way to the Foramen
1. See the downloadable PDF of this study at: http://rspb.royalsocietypublishing.org/content/279/1731/1161.full.pdf+html.
2. Haro Estroff Marano. "The Benefits of Laughter." *Psychology Today*, April 29, 2003. http://www.psychologytoday.com/articles/200304/the-benefits-laughter.

Chapter 15: Getting Your Marbles Back
1. Berchtold, N. C. & Cotman, C. W. "Evolution in the conceptualization of dementia and Alzheimer's disease: Greco-Roman period to the 1960s" *Neurobiology of Aging* (Vol. 19, 1998), 173–189.
2. *Nature Reviews Neurology* (Vol. 5, December 2009), 649-658.
3. Dr. Majid Fotuhi described his clinic's results in the book, *Boost Your Brain: The New Art and Science Behind Enhanced Brain Performance* (New York: HarperOne, 2013).
4. These tips provided by Dr. Majid Fotuhi, and used by permission.

Chapter 16: Brain Safe Your Home
1. "Clinical Guidance for Carbon Monoxide (CO) Poisoning After a Disaster," Centers for Disease Control and Prevention, http://emergency.cdc.gov/disasters/co_guidance.asp.
2. "Lead," Centers for Disease Control and Prevention, http://www.cdc.gov/nceh/lead/.
3. "Teenager Dies After Inhaling Dust-Off Cleaning Spray," http://urbanlegends.about.com/library/bl_dust_off.htm.
4. See: http://www.ncsu.edu/project/design-projects/udi/center-for-universal-design/the-principles-of-universal-design/.

Chapter 17: Eureka!
1. "University of Pittsburgh led study maps the making of a decision in the human brain," *Virtual Medical Worlds*, October 2007, http://www.hoise.com/vmw/07/articles/vmw/LV-VM-11-07-33.html.

Chapter 18: Feed Your Gold Mind
1. "MIT: Brain's Messengers Could Be Regulated-Potential For Better Understanding Of Schizophrenia," *Medical News Today*, September 17, 2007, http://www.medicalnewstoday.com/printerfriendlynews.php?newsid=82530.

Chapter 19: Don't Eat Squirrel Brains
1. Charles Wolfe, "Squirrel Brains May Be Unsafe," http://www.greysquirrel.net/brain.html.
2. Findings were published in *The Lancet* (350, no. 9078: August 30, 1997), http://www.mad-cow.org/~tom/victim23.html.
3. "Cow Brain Sandwiches Still on the Menu," http://www.rense.com/general47/still.htm.
4. "Prion," Wikipedia, http://en.wikipedia.org/wiki/Prion#cite_note-ictvdb-prions-29.
5. http://www.ncbi.nlm.nih.gov/pmc/articles/PMC2620635/.

Chapter 20: This is Your Brain on.... Any Questions?
1. A 2013 study of nearly 20,000 married couples in Norway found a high correlation between heavy drinking and divorce. See: http://www.sciencedaily.com/releases/2013/02/130205162519.htm.
2. www.nytimes.com/2013/02/05/science/brain-shape-may-play-role-in-cocaine-addiction. Accessed 5/14/2013.
3. www.drugabuse.gov/publlications/drugfacts/heroin. Accessed 5/4/2013.

Chapter 21: Stick to Quiet Fish
1. "Frequently Asked Questions About PCBs Found in Trout," http://www.fish.state.pa.us/qpcb2001.htm.
2. "What You Need to Know About Mercury in Fish and Shellfish," (US EPA: EPA-823-F-04-009).
3. "Is Fish Really Brain Food?" http://www.wellnessletter.com/html/wl/2001/wlFeatured1001.html.
4. The source of some of the information in this chapter is "The Smart Seafood Guide 2012," produced by www.foodandwaterwatch.org, and available for download at: http://www.foodandwaterwatch.org/fish/seafood/guide/.

Chapter 23: Participate by Proxy
1. "Sports Quotes," Thinkexist.com,http://thinkexist.com/quotations/sports/2.html.
2. "How Walking Buffs Your Brain," AARP, June, 2004, http://www.aarp.org/health/fitness/walking/a2004-06-04-walkingbrain.html.
3. "Playing, and Even Watching, Sports Improves Brain Function," *Science Daily*, September 3, 2008, http://www.sciencedaily.com/releases/2008/09/080901205631.htm.

4. Ibid.
5. Ibid.

Chapter 24: Fertilize Your Mind
1. "Heart health and lifestyle help seniors maintain brain power," February 22, 2006, http://www.newsmedical.net/news/2006/02/22/16130.aspx.
2. Bradley Hatfield, University of Maryland, College Park, School of Public Health, "Exercise Benefits Aging Brain, Alzheimer's," October 26, 2007, http://www.newsdesk.umd.edu/scitech/release.cfm?ArticleID=1532.
3. "Exercise in moderation best for the brain," *Medical Research News*, November 28, 2005, www.newsmedical.net/print_article.asp?id=14724.
4. From: "Exercise gives the brain a workout, too," CBS Evening News, January 30, 2009, www.cbsnews.com/stories/2009/01/30/earlyshow/health/main4764523.shtml.
5. See The Franklin Institute Resources for Science Learning, online article: http://www.fi.edu/learn/brain/exercise.html#physicalexercise.
6. C. Tudor-Locke, et al. "How many steps/day are enough?" *The International Journal of Behavioral Nutrition and Physical Activity* (July 28, 2011; 8:79. doi: 10.1186/1479-5868-8-79).

Chapter 25: Eat the Rainbow
1. "Coffee is number one source of antioxidants," Physorg.com, http://www.physorg.com/news6067.html.
2. "Higher Cognitive Performance with High Intake of Fruits and Vegetables," Elements4Health.com, http://www.elements4health.com/higher-cognitive-performancewith-high-intake-of-fruits-and-vegetables.html.
3. Original article: Denham Harman, "Aging: a theory based on free radical and radiation chemistry." *Journal of Gerontology* 11 (3):298–300. Theory summarized at: "Free radical theory of aging," Wikipedia, http://en.wikipedia.org/wiki/Free_radical_theory_of_aging.
4. Marlo Sollitto, "Power Foods: Doctors' Top Choices for Antioxidant Rich Foods," http://www.agingcare.com/Featured-Stories/113293/Power-Foods-Doctors-Top-Choices-for-Antioxidant-Rich-Foods.htm.
5. See the NIH report: http://nccam.nih.gov/health/antioxidants/introduction.htm.
6. "What's good for your heart is good for your head," Alz.org, http://www.alz.org/we_can_help_be_heart_smart.asp.
7. A more complete list is found at: http://kblog.lunchboxbunch.com/2010/02/eat-rainbow-colorfulfruits-and-veggies.html.

Chapter 26: Rot Not Thy Brain
1. "Couch potato," Answers.com, http://www.answers.com/topic/couch-potato.
2. Ibid.
3. Doc Gurley, "Is Your Brain a Couch Potato?" Sfgate.com, June 8, 2009, http://www.sfgate.com/cgibin/blogs/gurley/detail?entry_id=41335#ixzz0XXBeoiE3.
4. This quote and the adapted list of games at the end of this chapter can be found at: http://sharpbrains.com/resources/4-making-informed-brain-training-decisions/

description-highlights-and-validation-of-21-brain-training-products/. This additional study found more brain benefit from interactive online brain games, versus online crossword puzzles: http://online.wsj.com/article/PR-CO-20130501-913115.html?mod=googlenews_wsj.
5. Alvaro Fernandez and Dr. Elkhonon Goldberg, *The SharpBrains Guide to Brain Fitness* (San Francisco: SharpBrains, Inc., 2009), 8-9.

Chapter 27: You Can Go Home Again
1. From verse 2 of the hymn "Tell Me the Old, Old Story," lyrics by A. Katherine Hankey, 1866.
2. Terrence D. Hill, "Religion, Spirituality, and Healthy Cognitive Aging," *Southern Medical Journal* (99, no. 10, 2006): 1176-77.
3. Ibid.

Chapter 28: Stop and Smell the Memories
1. Diane Ackerman, *A Natural History of the Senses* (New York: Vintage Books, 1990), xv.
2. Ibid., 5.
3. "Loss of Smell Linked to Key Protein in Alzheimer's Disease," *Science Daily*, March 12, 2004, http://www.sciencedaily.com/releases/2004/03/040312090410.htm.
4. Study published by the University of Maryland Medical Center, "Parkinson's disease—Diagnosis," http://www.umm.edu/parkinsons/diagnosis.htm.
5. "Danger triangle of the face," Wikipedia, http://en.wikipedia.org/wiki/Danger_triangle_of_the_face.

Chapter 29: Can You Say, "Talafa Lava?"
1. J.W. King and Richard Suzman, "Prospects for Improving Cognition Throughout the Life Course," *Psychological Science in the Public Interest*, (vol. 9, no. 1, 2003): ii.
2. T. Kanaya, M. H. Scullin, and S. J. Ceci, "The Flynn Effect and U.S. Policies," *American Psychologist* (vol. 58, no. 10): 778–90.
3. Melonie Heron, et al, "Deaths: Final Data for 2006," *National Vital Statistics Reports* (57, no. 14, 2009).
4. S. Ge, C. Yang, K. Hsu, G. Ming, and H. Song, "A Critical Period of Enhanced Synaptic Plasticity In Newly Generated Neurons of the Adult Brain," *Neuron* (54, 2007): 559-66.

Chapter 30: "Water, Water Everywhere . . . Nor Any Drop to Drink"
1. "The Rime of the Ancient Mariner."
2. "Water, sanitation and hygiene links to health," World Health Organization: http://who.int/water_sanitation_health/publications/facts2004/en/print.html.
3. http://www.epa.gov/safewater/lead/pdfs.
4. Kathleen Doheny, "Bacteria May Lurk on Your Showerhead," http://www.webmd.com/lung/copd/news/20090914/bacteria-may-lurk-on-your-showerhead.
5. "Water Treatment Methods," Centers for Disease Control and Prevention, http://wwwnc.cdc.gov/travel/content/watertreatment.aspx.
6. "Lead in Paint, Dust, and Soil," U.S. EPA, http://www.epa.gov/lead/pubs/leadinfo.htm.

7. See the section on the pork tapeworm, in the chapter "Don't Eat Squirrel Brains." Other potential dangers to the brain from drinking untreated mountain water might involve ingesting contaminants from wild animals with central nervous system diseases.
8. "Healthy Swimming/Recreational Water," Centers for Disease Control and Prevention, http://www.cdc.gov/healthywater/swimming/index.html.
9. Matthew J. Kempton, et al. "Dehydration Affects Brain Structure and Function in Healthy Adolescents." *Human Brain Mapping*: 32:71-79 (2011).

Chapter 31: Cardiphonia

1. John Newton, *Cardiphonia* (Edinburgh, Scotland: Waugh and Innes, 1824), 74.
2. Free online access to this book can be found at: http://archive.org/details/cardiphoniaorthe00newtuoft.
3. Adapted from: Gary A. Burlingame, *Our God-Given Senses* (Orlando, FL: Healthy Life Press, 2013), 23.
4. As described by various sources, including online: http://ocarm.org/en/content/lectio/what-lectio-divina.
5. From Andrew Dreitcer, MDiv, PhD, at: http://www.patheos.com/Resources/Additional-Resources/Brain-on-God-Christian-Neuro-Spirituality.
6. Johnstone, B. and Glass, B. A. "Support for a Neuropsychological Model of Spirituality In Persons with Traumatic Brain Injury." *Journal of Religion and Science* (Volume 43, No. 4, 2008), 861–874.
7. Adapted from: http://www.fitbrains.com/brain-health/.

Chapter 32: Bug Off

1. Baz, P. D., *A Dictionary of Proverbs* (New York: Philosophical Library, Inc., 1963), 169.
2. CDC Lyme Disease Homepage, http://www.wrongdiagnosis.com/artic/cdc_lyme_disease_home_page_dvbid.htm.
3. "Insect repellents: which keep bugs at bay?" Consumer Reports, http://www.consumerreports.org/health/healthy-living/beauty-personal-care/personal-care/insect-repellents/insect-repellents-606/overview/index.htm.

Chapter 33: You are Hard Wired for Joy

1. "Single photon emission computed tomography," Wikipedia, http://en.wikipedia.org/wiki/Single_photon_emission_computed_tomography.
2. Earl Henslin, *This Is Your Brain on Joy* (Nashville: Thomas Nelson), 29.
3. Ibid., 39.
4. Ibid., 40.

Chapter 34: Where Past and Future Meet

1. "Memory," Quotegarden.com, http://www.quotegarden.com/memory.html. The Roadmender was a huge success in its time, and is available today online at: http://www.gutenberg.org/etext/705.
2. Ibid., 306.

3. Simakova, Mariya, "The Neurobiology of Nostalgia: A Story of Memory, Emotion, and the Self," Bryn Mawr College, 2002, http://serendip.brynmawr.edu/bb/neuro/neuro06/web3/msimakova.html.
4. "More Than Just Being a Sentimental Fool: The Psychology of Nostalgia," *Science Daily*, (December 14, 2008, http://www.sciencedaily.com/releases/2008/12/081212141851.htm.

Chapter 35: Buoy Your Amygdala
1. Mark Siegel, "The Irony of Fear," *The Washington Post*, August 30, 2005, http://www.washingtonpost.com/wp-dyn/content/article/2005/08/29/AR2005082901391.html.
2. Timothy Stokes, "Got a Stubborn Psychological Problem? You Can Probably Blame it on Your Amygdala," *Psychology Today*, September 14, 2009,
3. http://www.psychologytoday.com/blog/what-freud-didntknow/200909/got-stubborn-psychological-problem-you-can-probably-blame-your-amy.
4. Doug Holt, "The Role of the Amygdala in Fear and Panic," *SerendipUpdate*, January 8, 2008, http://serendip.brynmawr.edu/exchange/node/1749.

Chapter 36: The Secret of Your Senses
1. http://www.brainyquote.com/quotes/keywords/senses.html.
2. Aging Changes in the Senses," University of Maryland Medical Center (accessed February 19, 2009, http://www.umm.edu/ency/article/004013.htm.
3. Melissa Galea, "Brain Games," Alive (no. 297, July 2007), http://www.alive.com/6165a15a2.php?subject_bread_cramb=80.
4. Aging Changes in the Senses," *Alive* (no. 297, July 2007), http://www.alive.com/6165a15a2.php?subject_bread_cramb=80.
5. "Proprioception," The Sound Learning Centre, http://www.thesoundlearningcentre.co.uk/the-cause/proprioception-2/.

Chapter 37: Synaptic Serenades
1. "When Music Heals." Oliver Sacks, MD, Parade, March 31, 2002: http://www.bobjanuary.com/hhh/hhhpics/oliver.htm.
2. Daniel Levitin, *This is Your Brain on Music* (New York: Plume/Penguin, 2007), 227.
3. "Music for Babies, Music for Teenagers." Joshua Leeds, excerpted from *The Power of Sound* (Rochester, VT: Healing Arts Press, 2001). http://www.sound-remedies.com/musforbabmus.html.
4. See: http://arstechnica.com/science/2011/01/turns-out-that-music-really-is-intoxicating-after-all/; see also: http://sharpbrains.com/blog/2012/05/15/on-music-dopamine-and-making-sense-of-sound/ .
5. Sacks, "When Music Heals." http://www.bobjanuary.com/hhh/hhhpics/oliver.htm.
6. http://www.cnn.com/2013/04/15/health/brain-music-research. For information regarding the study see: http://www.cell.com/trends/cognitive-sciences/abstract/S1364-6613(13)00049-1.

Chapter 38: De-myth-ti-fying Brain Health
1. For more information, see: http://www.scientificamerican.com/article.cfm?id=strange-but-true-when-half-brain-better-than-whole, and http://hemifoundation.intuitwebsites. com/facts.html.
2. For more information, see: http://neurologyinstitute.com/.
3. http://www.fi.edu/learn/brain/stress.html.
4. See: http://www.nia.nih.gov/alzheimers/publication/alzheimers-disease-genetics-fact-sheet.
5. See: http://www.stanford.edu/group/hopes/cgibin/wordpress/2010/06/brain-derived-neurotrophic-factorbdnf/#can-exercising-promote-bdnf-production, and http://www.ninds.nih.gov/disorders/brain_basics/ninds_neuron.htm for more information.
6. http://online.wsj.com/article/SB10001424052970203935604577066293669642830.html?mod=WSJ_hp_MIDDLENexttoWhatsNewsFifth
7. http://med.emory.edu/ADRC/healthy_aging/healthy_aging/.
8. http://www.telegraph.co.uk/health/healthnews/7707157/Listening-to-Mozart-does-not-increase-intelligence.html.
9. The characteristics of a "gold standard" scientific "study" are that it be: **double-blind** (neither participants nor administrators know which subjects are getting the receiving the intervention); **placebo-controlled** (one group receives the intervention; a second group receives an inactive duplicate of the same intervention); and **randomized** (no one chooses which group a participant is in); conducted by **independent** researchers; and **published** in a peer-reviewed journal. Studies are even more reliable if they are: **cross-over** (when the groups switch and the one that got the intervention the first time now gets the placebo) where the results are the same; **duplicatable** (other researchers get the same results using the same methodology).

Chapter 39: Which Planet are You From?
1. John Gray, PhD. *Men are From Mars, Women are From Venus* (New York: Harper-Collins, 1993), xxx.
2. Elizabeth Heubeck,"How male and female brains differ: Researchers reveal sex differences in the brain's form and function." WebMD Feature, April 11, 2005. http://www.medicinenet.com/script/main/art.asp?articlekey=50512.
3. Walt & Barb Larimore, *His Brain, Her Brain* (Grand Rapids: Zondervan, 2008), 34.
4. Adapted from: http://www.amenclinics.com/dr-amen/latestnews/item/unleashing-the-power-of-the-female-brain. See Dr. Amen's book: *Unleash the Power of the Female Brain* for more on this subject.
5. Walt Larimore, MD, and Barb Larimore, *His Brain, Her Brain* (Grand Rapids: Zondervan, 2008), 81.

Chapter 40: Unfoggin' Your Noggin'
1. www.searchquotes.com/search/brain_fog/1/ Accessed 5/26/2013.
2. http://medical-dictionary.thefreedictionary.com/Brain+Fog Accessed 5/27/2013.
3. http://www.cleveland.com/healthfit/index.ssf/2013/03/moms_brain_fog_could_be_caused.html Accessed 5/27/2013.
4. http://www.lifescript.com/health/centers/fibromyalgia/articles/6_ways_to_beat_

fibro_fog.aspx. Accessed 5/27/2013.
5. C.S. Lewis, *A Grief Observed* (New York: HarperOne, 2009), 15.

Chapter 41: Toxic Shocks
1. http://gettingexback-howtowinyourexback.blogspot.com/2009/04/quotes-on-relationships.html.
2. These comments are adapted from: "Toxic Relationships: A Health Hazard." Sherrie Bourg Carter, PsyD, *Psychology Today*, August 7, 2011. http://www.psychologytoday.com/blog/high-octanewomen/201108/toxic-relationships-health-hazard.
3. "Toxic Stress: The Facts." Center on the Developing Child, Harvard University. http://developingchild.harvard.edu/topics/science_of_early_childhood/toxic_stress_response/.
4. "Overcome Toxic Emotions to Improve Your Relationships." Alberto Villoldo, PhD. Health and Wellness, January 27, 2011. http://www.sheknows.com/health-and-wellness/articles/823113/overcome-toxic-emotions-to-improve-your-relationships.
5. "Toxic Relationships Could Be Making You Ill.) Sun Meilan. Helium, January 29, 2012. http://www.helium.com/items/ 2285561-why-toxic-relationships-are-bad-for-you.
6. "Overcome Toxic Emotions to Improve Your Relationships." Alberto Villoldo, PhD. Health and Wellness, January 27, 2011. http://www.sheknows.com/health-and-wellness/articles/823113/overcome-toxic-emotions-to-improve-your-relationships.

Chapter 42: Unbind Your Mind
1. "Addiction Quotes," Great-Quotes.com, http://www.greatquotes.com/quotes/category/Addiction.htm.
2. "Questions and Answers on Addiction: 20-year brain-imaging program reveals clues about underlying mechanisms," Brookhaven National Laboratory: http://www.bnl.gov/bnlweb/PDF/Factsheet/FS_AddictionQA.pdf.
3. Michael Lemonick, "How We Get Addicted," Time, July 5, 2007, http://www.time.com/time/magazine/article/0,9171,1640436,00.html.
4. "Addiction and Brain Activity: What Happens in the Brain," Time, 2007, http://www.time.com/time/2007/addiction/.
5. Lemonick, op cit.
6. Engs, op cit.
7. Ibid.
8. Ibid.
9. Marnie C. Ferree. *No Stones*, (Xulon Press, 2002).
10. Heather Hatfield, "Shopping Spree, or Addiction?" WebMd, 2004, http://www.webmd.com/mental-health/features/shopping-spree-addiction.
11. Engs, op cit.
12. This list was created by the authors by comparing and combining information from various sources.

Chapter 43: This is Your Brain on Canvas
1. William H. Calvin, *The Throwing Madonna: Essays on the Brain* (New York: Bantam, 1991).
2. M. S. Gazzaniga, "Cerebral specialization and interhemispheric communication, Does the corpus callosum enable the human condition?" *Brain* (123: 7, 2000): 1293-1326.
3. T.M. Chamberlin Hodgson, B. Parris, M. James, N. Gutowski, M. Hussain, and C. Kennard, "The role of the ventral frontal cortex in inhibitory oculomotor control," *Brain* (130: 6, 2007): 1525-37.
4. Henry Ward Beecher, *Proverbs from Plymouth Pulpit*, 1887.

Chapter 44: Mind Your Head
1. "Traumatic brain injury (TBI) is the leading cause of death and disability in Americans under the age of 45. . . ." Lee, Hana, Max Wintermark, et al, "Focal Lesions in Acute Mile Traumatic Brain Injury and Neurocognitive Outcome: CT versus 3T MRI," *Journal of Neurotrauma* (September 25, 2008): 1049.
2. "Concussion," American Association of Neurological Surgeons, http://www.neurosurgerytoday.org/what/patient_e/concussion.asp.
3. "Study Links Concussions to Brain Disease," CBS News, http://www.cbsnews.com/stories/2009/10/09/60minutes/main5371686.shtml?tag=contentMain;cbsCarousel.
4. Numerous articles to this effect are posted online, including: http://www.bloomberg.com/news/2013-04-09/ex-nfl-players-lawyers-don-t-need-concussion-briefings.html.
5. "Concussion and Mild TBI," CDC, http://www.cdc.gov/concussion/.
6. "The Top 5 Causes of Head Injuries and How to Avoid Them," SixWise.com, http://www.sixwise.com/newsletters/05/09/28/the-top-5-causes-of-head-injuries-and-how-to-avoid-them.htm.
7. See: http://www.universaldesign.com/ for more information on Universal Design.
8. Ibid.
9. http://www.braintrauma.org/site/PageServer?pagename=TBI_Facts.
10. See: http://www.cdc.gov/traumaticbraininjury/statistics.html.

Chapter 45: Go Beltless
1. John Gullotta, "Taking Stock for Stroke Prevention, Australian Medical Association," Medical News Today, September 2008, www.medicalnewstoday.com/printerfriendlynews.php?newsid=121601.
2. "Stroke Facts and Statistics," CDC, http://www.cdc.gov/stroke/stroke_facts.htm.
3. Ibid.
4. Diana Rodriguez, "The 'Stroke Belt': Why Is Stroke Risk Higher in the Southeast?" http://www.everydayhealth.com/stroke/stroke-risk-higher-in-southeastern-us.aspx.
5. "Stroke Prevention," CDC, http://www.cdc.gov/stroke/prevention.htm.
6. "Cholesterol Control Plus Blood Pressure Control Equals Stroke Prevention," Medical News Today, April 2009, www.medicalnewstoday.com/printerfriendlynews.php?newsid=148273.

7. Egido, J.A., "Is psycho-physical stress a risk factor for stroke? A case-control study," *Journal of Neurology, Neurosurgery and Psychiatry*, Aug. 29, 2012.

Chapter 46: Listen to Your Other Brain
1. See: Thinkexist.com, http://www.thinkExist.com/quotes/with/keyword/gut.
2. "The Brain Gut Axis," http://www.ibsresearchupdate.org/IBS/brain1ie4.html.
3. Douglas Drossman, et al, "A Focus Group Assessment of Patients' Perspectives on Irritable Bowel Syndrome and Illness Severity," *Digestive Disease Science* (54, 7; July 2009): 1532-41.

Chapter 47: Reinvent Yourself
1. http://www.quotegarden.com/retirement.html.
2. Karla Freeman, "Don't Retire, Re-Invent!" My Article Archive, http://www.myarticlearchive.com/articles/7/176.htm.
3. Sue Poremba. "Another Shot: Reinventing Yourself After 60," *Grandparents Today*, http://www.grandparentstoday.com/articles/grandparent-leisure-time/another-shot-4421/.
4. Judy Shan Tsai Wendt, Robin Donnelly, Geert de Jong, and Farah Ahmed, "Age at retirement and long term survival of an industrial population: prospective cohort study," (Pub Med, 2005), http://www.pubmedcentral.nih.gov/articlerender.fcgi?artid=1273451.
5. Brian Kurth, "Reinventing Yourself After Retirement," Vocationvacations.com, http://vocationvacations.com/files/PDF/Reinventing_Yourself_After_Retirement.pdf.

Chapter 48: Play with Half a Glass
1. "Self-Talk," Great-Quotes.com, http://www.greatquotes.com/quotes/category/Self-Talk.htm.
2. The Dana Alliance for Brain Initiatives, *Staying Sharp: Learning as We Age* (New York: The Dana Alliance for Brain Initiatives, 2011), 19. See: http://www.dana.org/uploadedFiles/The_Dana_Alliances/Staying_Sharp/Staying%20Sharp%20Learning%20as%20We%20Age.pdf.
3. See: http://www.mayoclinic.com/health/positivethinking/SR00009.
4. From Philippians 4: *We've Got Mail, a Paraphrase of the New Testament Epistles* by Rev. Warren C. Biebel, *We've Got Mail* (Roseland, FL: Healthy Life Press, 2009), 58.
5. Martin Seligman, PhD, *Learned Optimism* (Vintage: New York, 2006), 224-225.

Chapter 49: Scrabble Your Brain
1. See: Thinkexist.com, http://thinkexist.com/quotes/with/keyword/game/2.html.
2. "Want to Improve Memory? Strengthen Your Synapses. Here's How," *Medical News Today* (January 2007), http://www.medicalnewstoday.com/articles/60455.php.
3. Ibid.
4. As quoted *The Wall Street Journal* article, posted online: http://online.wsj.com/article/SB10001424052970203458604577263273943183932.html.
5. These tips provided by Claire G. Herring, CEO and Chief Creative Officer, The

Rowing Team, LLC, and co-creator of: DaisyBrains.com and BlueOceanBrain.com.

Chapter 50: Welcome to Club Med
1. Source: http://www.agingcare.com/Articles/Polypharmacy-Dangerous-Drug-Interactions-119947.htm.
2. Campbell Noll, Malaz Boustani, Tony Limbil, et al, "Commonly Used Medications May Produce Cognitive Impairment in Seniors," Journal of Clinical Interventions in Aging (June 5, 2009).
3. Marc Ramirez, "More Die From Drugs Than Traffic Accidents," *The Seattle Times*, October 2, 2009, http://seattletimes.nwsource.com/cgi-bin/PrintStory.pl?document_id=2009985051&zsection.
4. Ibid.

Chapter 51: The Secret of Staying Focused
1. Adam J. Cox, "Understanding the Eight Pillars of Executive Control," http://concordspedpac.org/ExecutiveFunctions.html.
2. "Training Benefits Brains in Older People, Counters Aging Factors," Medical News Today, February 21, 2006, www.medicalnewstoday.com/printerfriendlynews.php?newsid=37973.
3. "Exercise keeps your brain from deteriorating," Medical News Today, October 18, 2008, http://www.medicalnewstoday.com/printerfriendlynews.php?newsid=125938.
4. This list is adapted from: "Executive Functions." http://en.wikipedia.org/wiki/Executive_functions.
5. Adam J. Cox, *No Mind Left Behind: Why Executive Control Skills are Essential for Every Child—and How Parents and Educators Can Sharpen Them* (Penguin Book Group, 2007).

Chapter 52: In Spirit and in Truth
1. Timothy R. Jennings, *Could It Be This Simple?* (Hagerstown, MD: Autumn House Publishing, 2007), 12.
2. See Acts 17:22 and the following verses to discover how Paul leveraged the religiousness of the Athenians.

Conclusion
1. For more information, see: http://www.rush.edu/rumc/page1099611542043.html.
2. For a list of published studies on this subject, see: http://www.positscience.com/why-brain-hq/world-classscience/peer-reviewed-research/published-scientific-studies.
3. http://www.psychologytoday.com/blog/heal-your-brain.
4. http://science.howstuffworks.com/life/isolation-effects.htm.
5. Dr. Paul Tournier was one of the first physicians to promote truly wholistic thinking in relation to patient care. He authored a number of books that anyone interested in this subject will find both helpful and meaningful, including: *A Place for You*; *The Meaning of Persons*; *To Understand Each Other*; *Guilt and Grace*; *Creative Suffering*; *The Gift of Feeling*; *Learning to Grow Old* and others.

Walt Larimore, MD, "Love Works Miracles" (© 2013).
1. Dr. Walt and Barb Larimore serve at Mission Medical Clinic in Colorado Springs, CO, and also serve on the Board of Life Network. Natives of Baton Rouge, LA, they have two adult children, two grandchildren, and an adopted tabby cat named Jack. Dr. Walt has written over two dozen books. Together, the Larimores authored the book *His Brain, Her Brain: How divinely designed differences can strengthen your marriage.*

Catalog of Resources   2015.01

Healthy Life Press

A Small, Independent Christian Publisher with a big mission—to help people live healthier lives physically, emotionally, spiritually, and relationally.

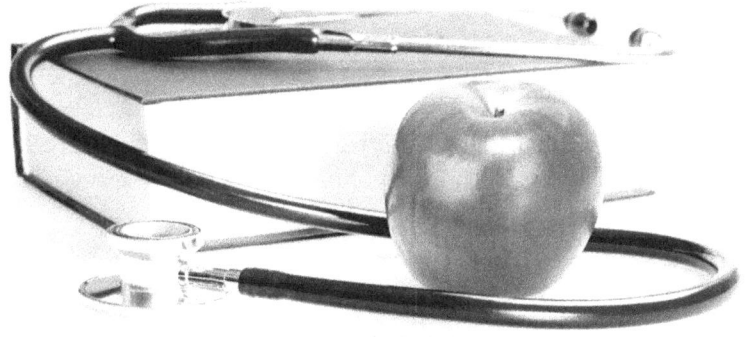

Golden, Colorado
www.healthylifepress.com
info@healthylifepress.com
1-877-331-2766

www.healthylifepress.com 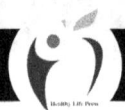 For information on our products, or how t publish with us, e-mail: *info@healthylifepress.*

I AM: Transformed in Him
A DVD Bible Study of the I AM Sayings
by Dianna Burg and Kim Tapfer

A six week DVD Bible study by women, for women.

Have you wanted a closer walk with the Lord? Do you sometimes find yourself dragging through your days wondering where he is, who he is, and why he isn't helping you more? In your heart of hearts, have you been hoping, perhaps even imagining, that God would reveal himself to you more and more, that he would help you to build a trust that would ease your burdens and, blessing of blessing, refashion your life into a grace- and peace-filled walk with him? Who does God say he is, and how can he answer these questions? In this DVD Bible study you will discover the deep and abiding riches of God, whose name is I AM WHO I AM, as he told Moses in the Book of Exodus. You will discover the many meanings and implications of each I AM saying from both an Old and New Testament perspective.

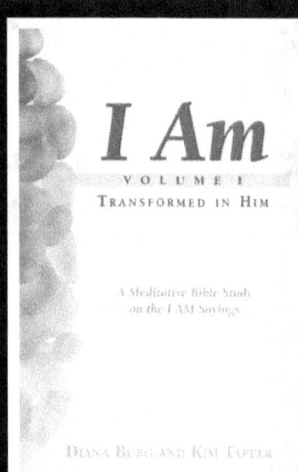

Paperback: $14.99   eBook: $9.99
Both: $19.99 (direct from publisher)

Stay Sharp
52 Ways to Keep Your Mind, Not Lose It
by Dr. David Biebel, James E. Dill, MD, and Bobbie Dill, RN

A once-a-week journey into the intricacies of the human —how it functions best, how to keep it healthy, how its health relates to your health in general, and the role of relationships and spirituality and other subjects not often discussed in a book on this subject.

Chapters are short, with practical tips offered following each. They are designed to stand alone, so you can focus on one per week if you wish, ignore some occasional informational overlap, and start anywhere you wish, because topics are arranged in no particular order.

This book will help you cut through the fog of hype and overstatement out there about brain health. And if you need hope in the face of a diagnosis of brain injury or brain disease in yourself or someone you love, this book is for you.

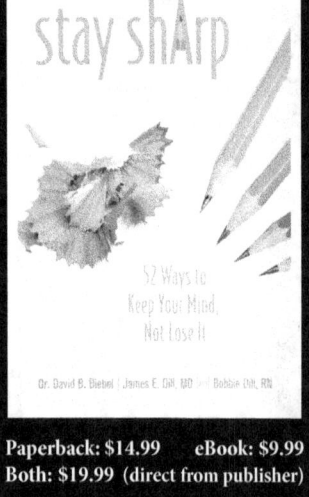

Paperback: $14.99   eBook: $9.99
Both: $19.99 (direct from publisher)

Printed books and eBooks available at
www.Amazon.com; *www.BN.com*;
www.deepershopping.com, and
wherever books are sold.

To order directly from the publisher,
visit: *www.healthylifepress.com*.
Unless otherwise noted on website, shipping
is free for all products purchased through HLP.

www.healthylifepress.com

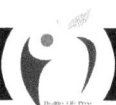

For information on our products, or how to publish with us, e-mail: *info@healthylifepress.com*

52 Ways to Feel Great Today
Once-a-Week Tips to Energize Your Life
by Dr. David Biebel, James E. Dill, MD, and Bobbie Dill, RN

This book demonstrates how changing your outlook can infuse your day with energy. You'll discover one creative yet simple, inexpensive, and fun thing for every week of the year. Chapters are short and succinct. Every suggestion is supported by at least one true story showing how implementing that idea was helpful to someone a lot like you. The stories are also included to encourage you to be as inventive, imaginative, playful, creative, or adventuresome as you can. *52 Ways to Feel Great Today* is not only based on the authors' experience and observations. Most of these "ways" have solid scientific evidence supporting their value in promoting your health and enhancing your happiness. Why settle for ordinary when you could be experiencing the extraordinary? "Good enough" can't be "good enough" when "great" is such a short stretch away. Reach for it today!

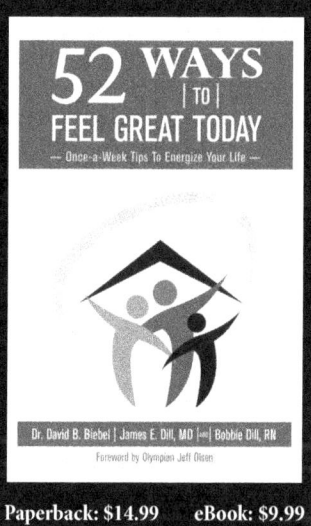

Paperback: $14.99   eBook: $9.99
Both: $19.99 (direct from publisher)

To Everything: A Season
by Dr. Herb Marlow

If you like mystery, danger, drama, romance, you will like this novel, the first in a new series to be published by Healthy Life Press. When Christian psychiatrist Dr. John Harlow returns to Grantsville, Nebraska, his sleepy hometown, he's hoping this homecoming will help him sort through the devastating sorrow of his past few months. Yes, he must settle the affairs of his recently deceased parents, including selling their home, the safest place of his youth. But this process proves easier than finding some sanctuary from his personal pain. Without really planning to do so, he sets up practice in Grantsville, only to find that the accoutrements of big city life have followed him home, including the psychological and spiritual maladies that seem rampant enough wherever you go. By the time he's done, Dr. Harlow has helped restore numerous relationships, solved a murder mystery, and heroically saved more than one life. Yet in the process he's left himself, and those he's recently come to love, at risk from terrorists driven by hatred and revenge at any cost.

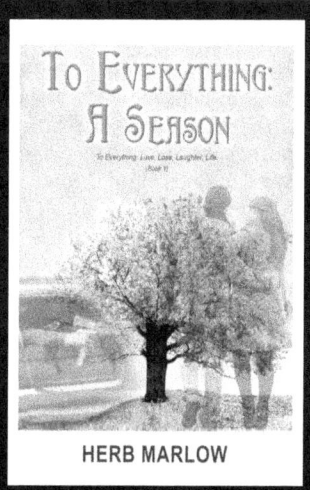

Paperback: $14.99   eBook: $9.99
Both: $19.99 (direct from publisher)

Printed books and eBooks available at
www.Amazon.com; *www.BN.com*;
www.deepershopping.com, and
wherever books are sold.

To order directly from the publisher,
visit: *www.healthylifepress.com*.
Unless otherwise noted on website, shipping
is free for all products purchased through HLP.

www.healthylifepress.com

For information on our products, or how to publish with us, e-mail: *info@healthylifepress.com*

A Hole in the Fence
Getting to the Other Side of Divorce
by Lynn Carroll

Carroll peels back the layers of the divorce experience like an onion, while sharing how the she discovered that with every emotion and circumstance God was present. Using the "hole in the fence" to picture the process of divorce, she describes how some people led the way to the other side; some walked beside and took her hand; and how at the most difficult times she was carried through by God. This book examines the emotions of divorce from A-Z literally. Through anecdote, story, poetry, and expert advice, each emotion is described, with positive and negative responses matched. For example, there's "Anger – Abundance" and "Betrayal – Beauty" and "Depression – Discovery." Because of this unique organization, readers can begin with a section that connects closely with their current experience, and then move on to others.

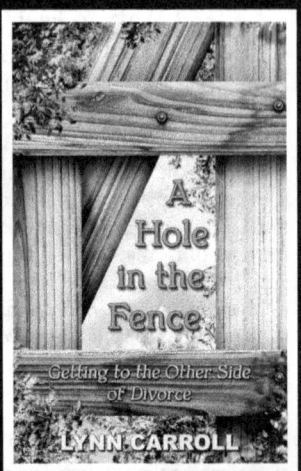

Paperback: $14.99   eBook: $9.99
Both: $19.99 (direct from publisher)

Our Favorite Verses
Once-a-Week Tips to Energize Your Life
compiled and edited by Tina Ware-Walters, PhD

A collection of "favorite" Scripture passages from nearly thirty contributors who share their stories of how the Word of God helped them in some very practical way. It is a veritable smorgasbord for your soul. And it's organized to match the need of your moment. For example, when you're so pressed that you only have time for some fast food, you can snack on a short devotional from the "Quick Inspiration" section. Or perhaps today you could really use a recipe for converting those unsavory challenges into something more palatable, in which case a small adjustment in "Perspective," might prove invaluable. Or maybe you need a generous serving of encouragement from learning how people a lot like you have faced difficulties a lot like yours, emboldened, strengthened, and sustained by their favorite verses of "Comfort" from the Word of God.

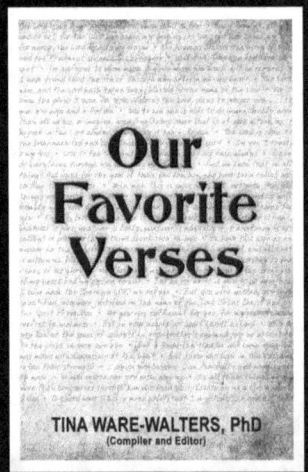

Paperback: $12.99   eBook: $9.99
Both: $17.99 (direct from publisher)

Printed books and eBooks available at
www.Amazon.com; *www.BN.com*;
www.deepershopping.com, and
wherever books are sold.

To order directly from the publisher,
visit: *www.healthylifepress.com*.
Unless otherwise noted on website, shipping
is free for all products purchased through HLP.

www.healthylifepress.com

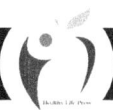

For information on our products, or how to publish with us, e-mail: *info@healthylifepress.com*

Tricky Ricky
The Homestead Twins (Part 1)
by Jannis Hibberts

The first in a series of stories featuring the twins, Richard and Rachel, who live there with their parents, Mama and Papa. The twins are home schooled, and they live in the fertile and beautiful Pacific Northwest of the United States. They help their parents cultivate and care for their little farm so it produces most of the food the family needs, all year round. When they're not studying or helping with the homestead, the twins have many adventures in which they invite you to join them, like the one described in this book.

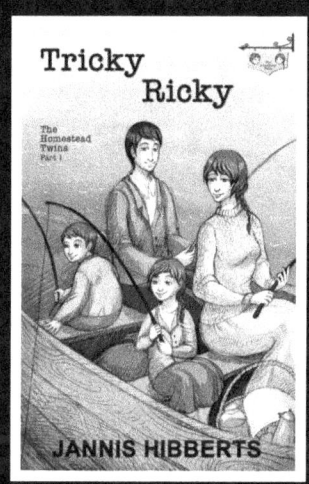

Paperback: $12.99   eBook: $9.99
Both: $17.99 (direct from publisher)

Mommy, What's 'Died' Mean?
How the Butterfly Story Helped Little Dave Understand His Grandpa's Death
by Linda Swain Gill
illustrated by David Lee Bass (a.k.a. "Little Dave")

Designed to assist Christian parents and other adults who love and care about children to talk with them about the difficult subject of death, the story traces a small child's experience following his grandpa's and shows how his mother sensitively answered his questions about death by using simple examples derived from the birth of a butterfly. Little Dave's story is colorfully illustrated and designed for a child and parent or trusted adult to read together. The story has been created especially for children from pre-kindergarten through 4th grade. Discussion questions are included for each story page to help determine how much the child understands. A simple imitation game is also included to help involve the child in the story. Several pages at the end of the book contain suggestions about how to discuss death and dying with children of various ages.

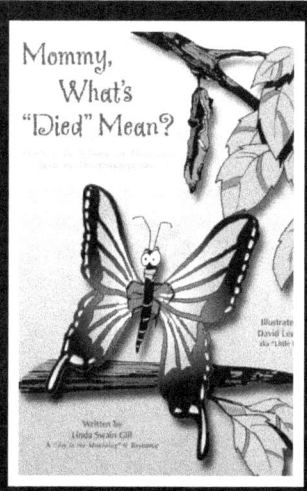

Paperback: $14.99   eBook: $9.99
Both: $19.99 (direct from publisher)

Printed books and eBooks available at
www.Amazon.com; *www.BN.com*;
www.deepershopping.com, and
wherever books are sold.

To order directly from the publisher,
visit: *www.healthylifepress.com*.
Unless otherwise noted on website, shipping
is free for all products purchased through HLP.

www.healthylifepress.com

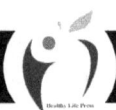

For information on our products, or how to publish with us, e-mail: *info@healthylifepress.com*

No Worries
Spiritual and Mental Health Counseling for Anxiety
by Elaine Leong Eng, MD

Offering a unique spiritual and mental health perspective on a major malady of our age, this practicing Christian psychiatrist has packed a dose of reality mixed with medicine and faith into a book aimed at informing, inspiring, and equipping those who wish to better help those who struggle with anxiety and related disorders, both inside and outside the church. As one endorser said, "I travel all over the world. I see fellow believers suffering from different forms of anxiety and worry. Dr. Eng's book gives me tools to recognize when people are suffering and how to encourage them to get the help they need."

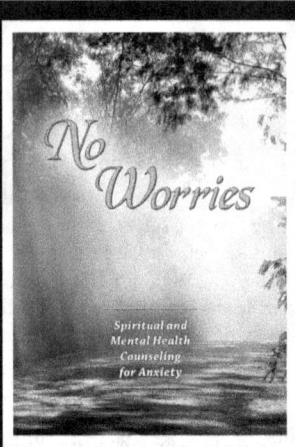

Paperback: $19.99   eBook: $9.99
Both: $24.99 (direct from publisher)

If God is So Good, Why Do I Hurt So Bad?
by David B. Biebel, DMin

This **25th Anniversary Edition** of a best-selling classic (over 200,000 copies in print worldwide, in a dozen languages) is the book's first major revision since its initial release in 1989. This new version features additional original material related to the conundrum of suffering and faith (with principles learned along the way), and chapter ending questions for personal or group use.

Endorser Sheila Walsh wrote, "*I believe this is one of the most profound, empathetic and beautiful books ever written on the subject of suffering and loss. There is no attempt to quickly ease our pain but rather, with an understanding born in the crucible God uniquely designed for him, David offers a place to stand, a place to fall and a place to rise again. This book left an indelible mark on my heart over twenty years ago and now with this new release the gift is fresh and fragrant. I highly commend this to you!*"

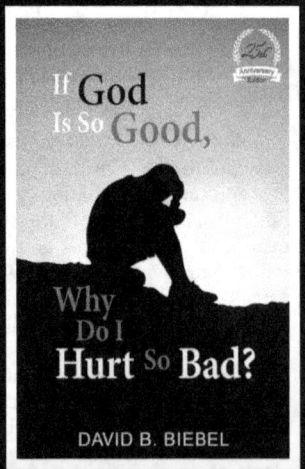

Paperback: $14.99   eBook: $9.99
Both: $19.99 (direct from publisher)

Printed books and eBooks available at
www.Amazon.com; *www.BN.com*;
www.deepershopping.com, and
wherever books are sold.

To order directly from the publisher,
visit: *www.healthylifepress.com*.
Unless otherwise noted on website, shipping
is free for all products purchased through HLP.

www.healthylifepress.com

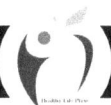

For information on our products, or how to publish with us, e-mail: *info@healthylifepress.com*

We've Got Mail
The New Testament Letters in Modern English As Relevant Today as Ever!
by Rev. Warren C. Biebel, Jr.

A modern English paraphrase of the New Testament Letters, sure to inspire in readers a loving appreciation for God's Word.

Warren Biebel's pastoral interpretation of the New Testament letters is a highly readable and enjoyable re-write of a large portion of the New Testament. Biebel makes it clear that, while his work is not a word-for-word translation of these letters, he tries to stay true to the apparent meaning of the text. He has done a good job of making some difficult passages more readable, and the delight that comes from reading this book increases one's desire to understand and apply the principles and doctrines about which the authors wrote. My hope is that this work will take its place as a strong paraphrase—among such greats as "Living Letters" and "The Message."
– David Wickstrom, PhD

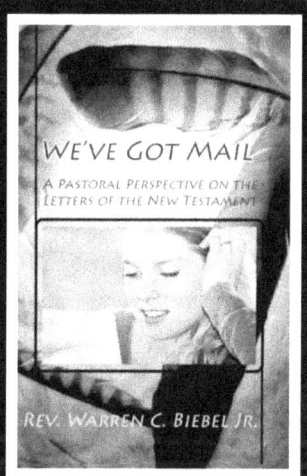

Paperback: $9.99   eBook: $6.99
Both: $14.99 (direct from publisher)

Who Me, Pray?
Prayer 101: Praying Aloud, for Beginners
by Gary A. Burlingame

Who Me, Pray? is a practical guide for prayer, based on Jesus' direction in "The Lord's Prayer," with examples provided for use in typical situations where you might be asked or expected to pray in public.

If Jesus is our friend, then why don't we talk with Him more often? Perhaps it is because prayer as practiced by many Christians is a cold exercise rather than a warm conversation. Who me, pray? is a simple, down-to-earth guide that will help the ordinary Christian learn to talk with God in prayer. I recommend it.
– Eric Wallace
President, Institute for Uniting Church and Home

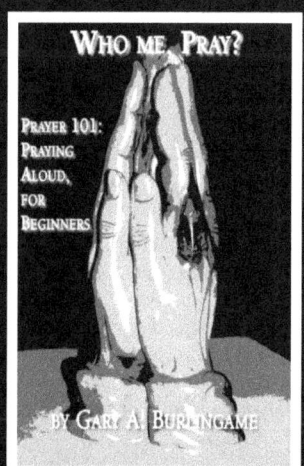

Paperback: $6.99   eBook: $2.99
Both: $7.99 (direct from publisher)

Printed books and eBooks available at
www.Amazon.com; *www.BN.com*;
www.deepershopping.com, and
wherever books are sold.

To order directly from the publisher,
visit: *www.healthylifepress.com*.
Unless otherwise noted on website, shipping
is free for all products purchased through HLP.

www.healthylifepress.com

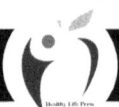

For information on our products, or how to publish with us, e-mail: info@healthylifepress.com

My Broken Heart Sings
The Poetry of Gary Burlingame
by Gary A. Burlingame

In 1987, Gary and his wife Debbie lost their son Christopher John, at only six months of age, to a chronic lung disease. This life-changing experience gave them a special heart for helping others through similar loss and pain.

Gary Burlingame's poetry has been on display in my waiting room for many years. His poems have touched the lives of many patients and their families. His poems stir the emotions while being practical, insightful, spiritual, and deeply truthful. I am glad to have his poetry in book form to refer to my patients and friends for support when they find themselves in pain and fall into deep struggles in their own lives.

– David Trumbore, PhD

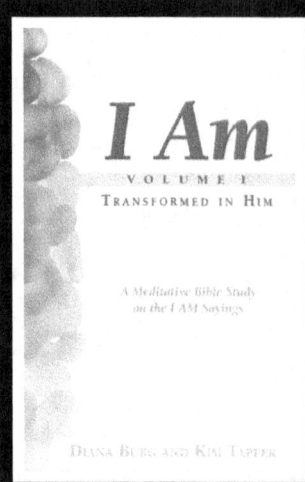

Paperback: $10.99   eBook: $6.99
Both: $13.99 (direct from publisher)

After Normal
One Teen's Journey Following Her Brother's Death
by Diane Aggen

Based on a journal the author kept following her younger brother's death. It offers helpful insights and understanding for teens facing a similar loss or for those who might wish to understand and help teens facing a similar loss.

Honest, insightful, real . . . After Normal is a most helpful look inside the heart of a teen-age girl trying to find her way after the death of her younger brother. I heartily recommend this book for anyone on a similar journey, and for those who wish to understand how that unique pain really feels.

– Jo Marturano, MD, Psychiatrist

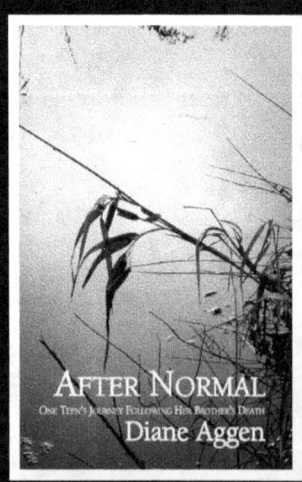

Paperback: $11.99   eBook: $6.99
Both: $14.99 (direct from publisher)

Printed books and eBooks available at
www.Amazon.com; www.BN.com;
www.deepershopping.com, and
wherever books are sold.

To order directly from the publisher,
visit: www.healthylifepress.com.
Unless otherwise noted on website, shipping
is free for all products purchased through HLP.

www.healthylifepress.com

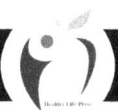

For information on our products, or how to publish with us, e-mail: *info@healthylifepress.com*

In the Unlikely Event of a Water Landing
Lessons Learned from Landing in the Hudson River
by Andrew Jamison, MD

The author was flying standby on US Airways Flight 1549 toward Charlotte on January 15, 2009, from New York City, where he had been interviewing for a residency position. Little did he know that the next stop would be the Hudson River. Riveting and inspirational, this book would be especially helpful for people in need of hope and encouragement.

When the chips are down one's character will find expression, one way or another.

– David Stevens, MD
CEO, Christian Medical
& Dental Associations

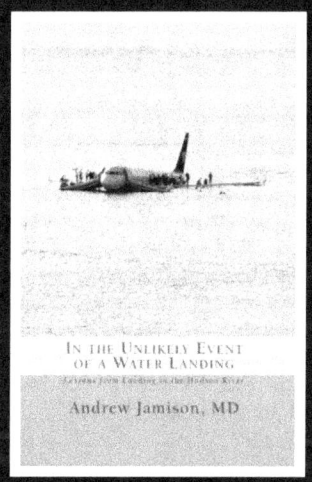

Paperback: $8.99   eBook: $6.99
Both: $12.99 (direct from publisher)

Finding Martians in the Dark
Everything I Needed to Know About Teaching Took Me Only 30 Years to Learn
by Dan M. Biebel

Packed with wise advice based on hard experience, and laced with humor, this book is a perfect teacher's gift year-round. Susan J. Wegmann, PhD, says, "Biebel's sardonic wit is mellowed by a genuine love for kids and teaching. . . . A Whitman-like sensibility flows through his stories of teaching, learning, and life."

A wonderful book. Honest and heartfelt, practical and wise, it embeds lessons of teaching and learning in a rich set of personal accounts.

– Tom Schram, PhD
University of New Hampshire

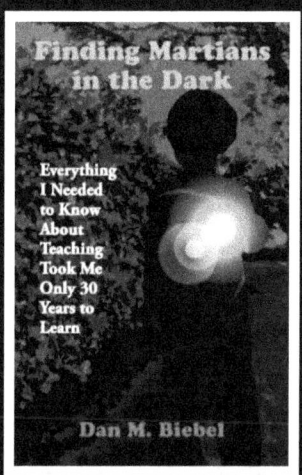

Paperback: $10.99   eBook: $6.99
Both: $14.99 (direct from publisher)

Printed books and eBooks available at
www.Amazon.com; www.BN.com;
www.deepershopping.com, and
wherever books are sold.

To order directly from the publisher,
visit: *www.healthylifepress.com*.
Unless otherwise noted on website, shipping
is free for all products purchased through HLP.

www.healthylifepress.com

For information on our products, or how to publish with us, e-mail: *info@healthylifepress.com*

Because We're Family
and
Because We're Friends
by Gary A. Burlingame

Sometimes things related to faith can be hard to discuss with your family and friends. These booklets are designed to be given as gifts, to help you open the door to discussing spiritual matters with family members and friends who are open to such a conversation.

From the books:
Far too often we avoid having difficult discussions with people we care about. Let's not let that happen between us.

Paperback: $5.99 ea
eBook: $4.99 ea.
Both (of same title): $9.99
(direct from publisher)

Paperback: $5.99 ea
eBook: $4.99 ea.
Both (of same title): $9.99
(direct from publisher)

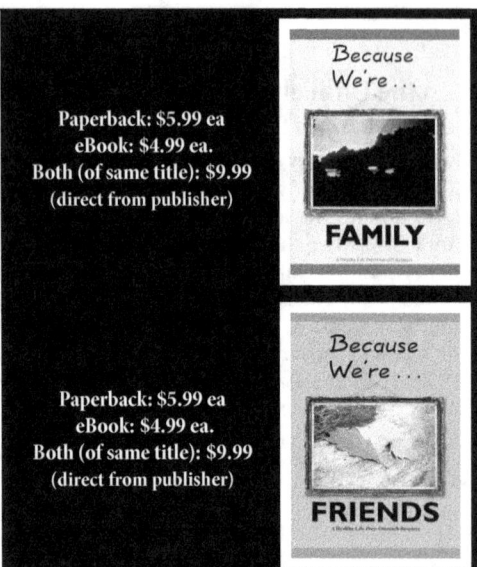

The Transforming Power of Story
Telling Your Story Brings Hope to Others and Healing to Yourself
by Elain Leong Eng, MD and David B. Biebel, DMin

This book demonstrates, through multiple true life stories, how sharing one's story, especially in a group setting, can bring hope to listeners and healing to the one who shares. Individuals facing difficulties will find this book greatly encouraging.

Dr. Elaine Eng is a remarkable woman with an incredible story and personal ministry. She has been an inspiration to me for as long as I have known her. Her book will inspire you, bring tears of joy to your eyes, and longing to your heart, and reinforce your love for our wonderful Savior. Dr. Eng is a living, walking testimony to God's grace and power through human frailty. Her life and her stories show poignantly how He can use any circumstance for His glory.

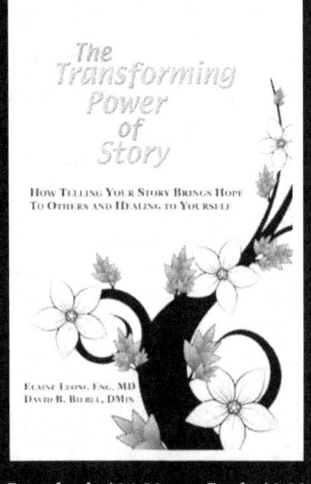

Paperback: $14.99   eBook: $9.99
Both: $19.99 (direct from publisher)

Printed books and eBooks available at
www.Amazon.com; *www.BN.com*;
www.deepershopping.com, and
wherever books are sold.

To order directly from the publisher,
visit: *www.healthylifepress.com*.
Unless otherwise noted on website, shipping is free for all products purchased through HLP.

www.healthylifepress.com 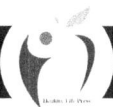 For information on our products, or how to publish with us, e-mail: *info@healthylifepress.com*

You Deserved a Better Father
Good Parenting Takes a Plan
by Robb Brandt, MD

About parenting by intention, and other lessons the author learned through the loss of his firstborn son. It is especially for parents who believe that bits and pieces of leftover time will be enough for their own children.

A compelling case for intentional fatherhood and an encouragement for parents to seize the moments with their kids. I recommend it."
— Rick Santorum, Former United States Senator and Chairman of the Senate Republican Conference

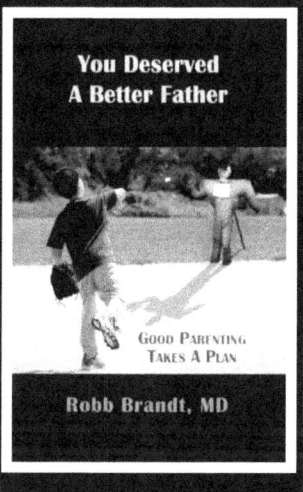

Paperback: $12.99   eBook: $6.99
Both: $17.99 (direct from publisher)

Jonathan, You Left Too Soon
by David B. Biebel, DMin

One pastor's journey through the loss of his son, into the darkness of depression, and back into the light of joy again, emerging with a renewed sense of mission.

Not since Joe Bayly's A View from the Hearse *have I found myself more in agreement. To this author, grief is real; it dare not be denied or ignored. Yes, its wounds must be handled with care and given time to heal. Preserving us from pious platitudes and empty clichés, David Biebel says it straight and he says it well. Best of all, he doesn't attempt to answer all the whys.*
— Charles Swindoll

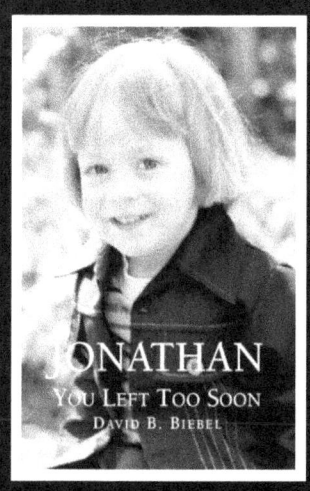

Paperback: $12.99   eBook: $5.99
Both: $14.99 (direct from publisher)

Printed books and eBooks available at
www.Amazon.com; www.BN.com;
www.deepershopping.com, and
wherever books are sold.

To order directly from the publisher,
visit: *www.healthylifepress.com*.
Unless otherwise noted on website, shipping
is free for all products purchased through HLP.

www.healthylifepress.com

For information on our products, or how to publish with us, e-mail: *info@healthylifepress.c*

The Spiritual Fitness Checkup
for the 50-Something Woman
by Sharon V. King, PhD

Following the stages of a routine medical exam, the author describes ten spiritual fitness "checkups" midlife women can conduct to assess their spiritual health and tone up their relationship with God. Each checkup consists of the author's personal reflections, a Scripture reference for meditation, and a "Spiritual Pulse Check," with exercises readers can use for personal application.

The Spiritual Fitness Checkup for the 50-something Woman is your guide to toning up your relationship with God at your midlife milepost. This book is for you if:
- You had 50 or more candles on your last birthday cake.
- You think "fitness" is all about getting skinny.
- Your spiritual life is important to you.

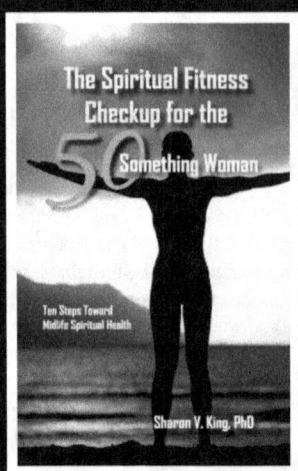

Paperback: $8.99   eBook: $6.99
Both: $12.99 (direct from publisher)

The Other Side of Life
Over 60? God Still Has a Plan for You
by Rev. Warren C. Biebel, Jr.

Drawing on biblical examples and his 60-plus years of pastoral experience, Rev. Biebel helps older (and younger) adults understand God's view of aging and the rich life available to everyone who seeks a deeper relationship with God as they age. Rev. Biebel explains how to: Identify God's ongoing plan for your life; Rely on faith to manage the anxieties of aging; Form positive, supportive relationships; Cultivate patience; Cope with new technologies; Develop spiritual integrity; Understand the effects of dementia; Develop a Christ-centered perspective of aging.

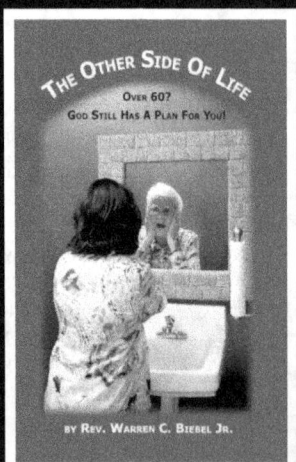

Paperback: $10.99   eBook: $6.99
Both: $14.99 (direct from publisher)

Printed books and eBooks available at
www.Amazon.com; *www.BN.com*;
www.deepershopping.com, and
wherever books are sold.

To order directly from the publisher,
visit: *www.healthylifepress.com*.
Unless otherwise noted on website, shipping
is free for all products purchased through HLP.

www.healthylifepress.com

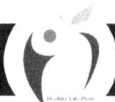

For information on our products, or how to publish with us, e-mail: *info@healthylifepress.com*

My Faith, My Poetry
by Gary A. Burlingame

This unique book of Christian poetry is actually two in one. The first collection of poems, A Day in the Life, explores a working parent's daily journey of faith. The reader is carried from morning to bedtime, from "In the Details," to "I Forgot to Pray," back to "Home Base," and finally to "Eternal Love Divine." The second collection of poems, Come Running, is wonder, joy, and faith wrapped up in words that encourage and inspire the mind and the heart.

I carry your book in my work bag and I have a great time picking out "my favorites." By the time I read it again I'll have more "favorites." They are all very good and on target. Aside from the actual poetry writing (inspired), your layout and cover are so pleasing to the eye. A beautiful presentation!!

– Christian author, Philadelphia

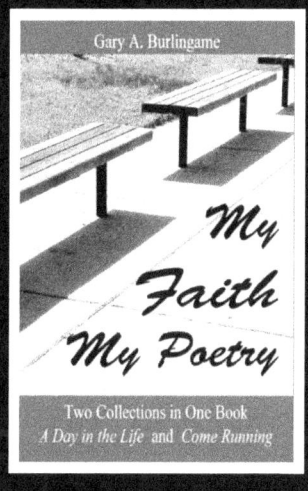

Paperback: $10.99   eBook: $6.99
Both: $13.99 (direct from publisher)

On Eagles' Wings
by Sara Eggleston

One woman's life journey from idyllic through chaotic to joy, carried all the way by the One who has promised to never leave us nor forsake us. Remarkable, poignant, moving, and inspiring, this autobiographical account will help many who are facing difficulties that seem too great to overcome or even bear at all. It is proof that Isaiah 40:31 is as true today as when it was penned, "But they that wait upon the LORD shall renew their strength; they shall mount up with wings as eagles; they shall run, and not be weary; and they shall walk, and not faint."

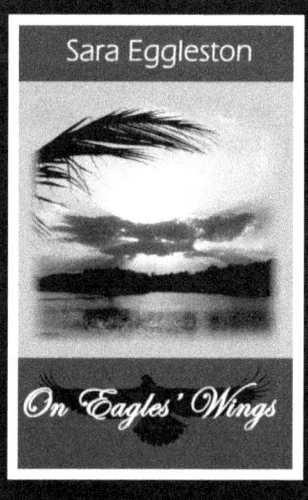

Paperback: $14.99   eBook: $8.99
Both: $22.99 (direct from publisher)

Printed books and eBooks available at
www.Amazon.com; *www.BN.com*;
www.deepershopping.com, and
wherever books are sold.

To order directly from the publisher,
visit: *www.healthylifepress.com*.
Unless otherwise noted on website, shipping
is free for all products purchased through HLP.

www.healthylifepress.com

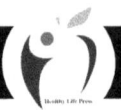

For information on our products, or how to publish with us, e-mail: *info@healthylifepress.com*

Richer Descriptions
by Gary A. Burlingame

A unique manual that explores all nine human senses in seven chapters for use by Christian speakers and writers. Applications are encouraged by exercises, a speaker's checklist, writing samples, and a writer's guide. Bible references encourage a deeper appreciation of being created by God for a sensory experience. The common senses of smell, taste, touch, sight, and hearing are covered as well as thermoception, nociception, equilibrioception, and the kinesthetic sense.

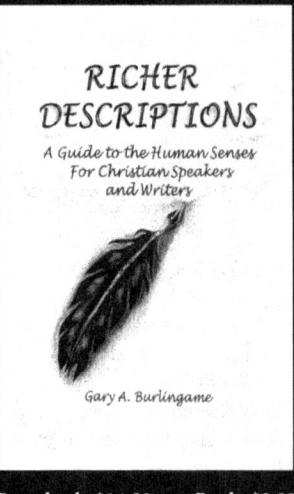

Paperback: $14.99   eBook: $8.99
Both: $22.99 (direct from publisher)

Treasuring Grace
by Rob Plumley and Tracy Roberts

This novel was inspired by a dream. Liz Swanson's life isn't quite what she'd imagined, but she considers herself lucky. She has a good husband, beautiful children, and fulfillment outside of her home through volunteer work. On some days she doesn't even notice the dull ache in her heart. While she's preparing for their summer kickoff at Lake George, the ache disappears and her sudden happiness is mistaken for anticipation of their weekend. However, as the family heads north, there are clouds on the horizon that have nothing to do with the weather. Only Liz's daughter, who's found some of her mother's hidden journals, has any idea what's wrong. But by the end of the weekend, there will be no escaping the truth or its painful buried secrets.

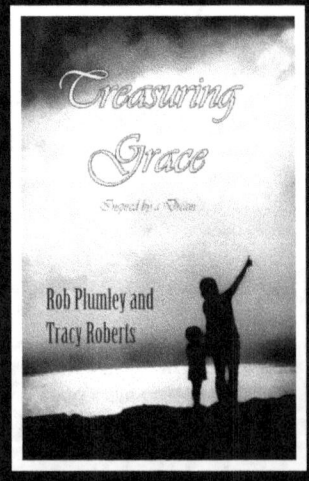

Paperback: $12.99   eBook: $7.99
Both: $19.99 (direct from publisher)

Printed books and eBooks available at
www.Amazon.com; www.BN.com;
www.deepershopping.com, and
wherever books are sold.

To order directly from the publisher,
visit: *www.healthylifepress.com*.
Unless otherwise noted on website, shipping
is free for all products purchased through HLP.

www.healthylifepress.com

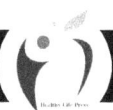

For information on our products, or how to publish with us, e-mail: *info@healthylifepress.com*

From Orphan to Physician
The Winding Path
by Chun-Wai Chan, MD

From the foreword: "In this book, Dr. Chan describes how his family escaped to Hong Kong, how they survived in utter poverty, and how he went from being an orphan to graduating from Harvard Medical School and becoming a cardiologist. The writing is fluent, easy to read and understand. The sequence of events is realistic, emotionally moving, spiritually touching, heart-warming, and thought provoking. The book illustrates . . . how one must have faith in order to walk through life's winding path."

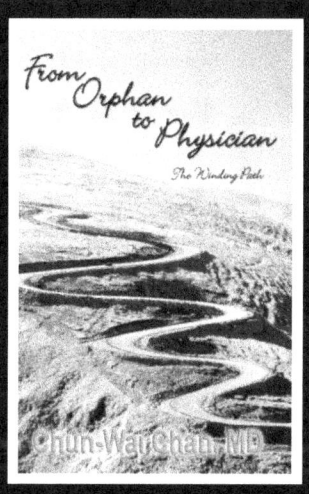

Paperback: $14.99   eBook: $8.99
Both: $22.99 (direct from publisher)

12 Parables
by Wayne Faust

Timeless Christian stories about doubt, fear, change, grief, and more. Using tight, entertaining prose, professional musician and comedy performer Wayne Faust manages to deal with difficult concepts in a simple, straightforward way. These are stories you can read aloud over and over—to your spouse, your family, or in a group setting. Packed with emotion and just enough mystery to keep you wondering, while providing lots of points to ponder and discuss when you're through, these stories relate the gospel in the tradition of the greatest speaker of parables the world has ever known, who appears in them often.

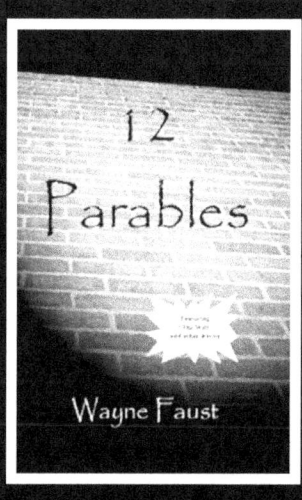

Paperback: $14.99   eBook: $9.99
Both: $19.99 (direct from publisher)

Printed books and eBooks available at
www.Amazon.com; *www.BN.com*;
www.deepershopping.com, and
wherever books are sold.

To order directly from the publisher,
visit: *www.healthylifepress.com*.
Unless otherwise noted on website, shipping
is free for all products purchased through HLP.

www.healthylifepress.com

For information on our products, or how to publish with us, e-mail: info@healthylifepress.c

The Answer is Always "Jesus"
by Aram Haroutunian

Written by a pastor who gave children's sermons for 15 years at a large church in Golden, Colorado—well over 500 in all. This book contains 74 of his most unforgettable presentations—due to the children's responses. Pastors, homeschoolers, parents who often lead family devotions, or other storytellers will find these stories, along with comments about props and how to prepare and present them, an invaluable asset in reconnecting with the simplest, most profound truths of Scripture, and then to envision how best to communicate these so even a child can understand them.

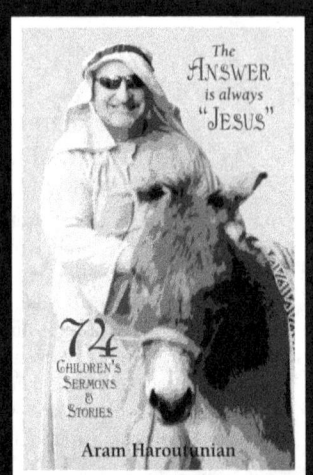

Paperback: $12.99   eBook: $8.99
Both: $19.99 (direct from publisher)

Handbook of Faith
by Rev. Warren C. Biebel, Jr.

The New York Times World 2011 Almanac claimed that there are 2 billion, 200 thousand Christians in the world, with "Christians" being defined as "followers of Christ." The original 12 followers of Christ changed the world; indeed, they changed the history of the world. So this author, a pastor with over 60 years' experience, poses and answers this logical question: "If there are so many 'Christians' on this planet, why are they so relatively ineffective in serving the One they claim to follow?" Answer: Because, unlike Him, they do not know and trust the Scriptures, implicitly. This little volume will help you do that.

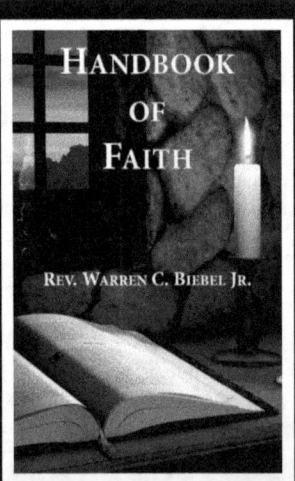

Paperback: $8.99   eBook: $6.99
Both: $13.99 (direct from publisher)

Printed books and eBooks available at
www.Amazon.com; www.BN.com;
www.deepershopping.com, and
wherever books are sold.

To order directly from the publisher,
visit: www.healthylifepress.com.
Unless otherwise noted on website, shipping
is free for all products purchased through HLP.

www.healthylifepress.com

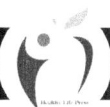

For information on our products, or how to publish with us, e-mail: *info@healthylifepress.com*

Pieces of My Heart
by David L. Wood

Eighty-two lessons from normal everyday life. David's hope is that these stories will spark thoughts about God's constant involvement and intervention in our lives and stir a sense of how much He cares about every detail that is important to us.

The front cover is symbolic of my children, for whom this book was written. They are all loved and cherished in my heart and therefore, each one is represented by a piece of my heart. The missing piece of the heart and the butterfly flying overhead are symbolic of my son, Daniel, who died shortly before his first birthday. Losing Daniel was the hardest thing I have faced in this life and he took a piece of my heart with him to heaven when he left. The butterfly is flying toward the sun, which is a representation of God and our eternal life to come. On the back cover, there is a lighthouse. This lighthouse is Jesus, who leads us and guides us through this wild ride we call 'life.'

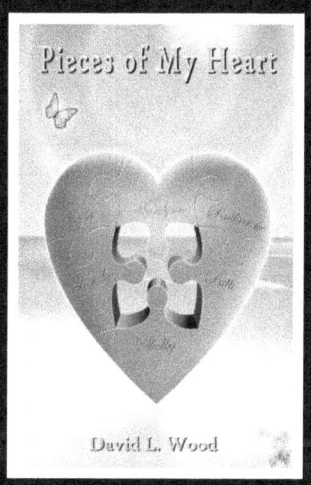

Paperback: $16.99   eBook: $8.99
Both: $24.99 (direct from publisher)

Dream House
by Justa Carpenter

Written by a New England builder of several hundred homes, the idea for this book came to him one day as he was driving from one job site to another. He pulled over and recorded it so he would remember it, and now you will remember it, too, if you believe, as he does, that ". . . He who has begun a good work in you will complete it until the day of Jesus Christ."

One of the greatest challenges of the Christian life is to give ourselves entirely to God and trust Him to build our lives and our characters exactly as He wants us to be, even if the process does not take the path that we would prefer.

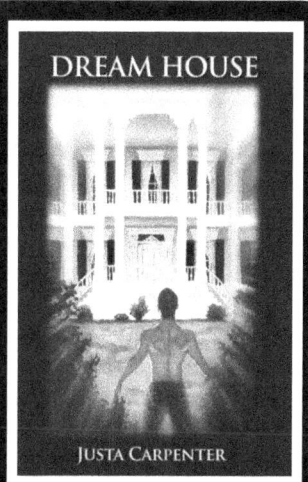

Paperback: $10.99   eBook: $6.99
Both: $13.99 (direct from publisher)

Printed books and eBooks available at
www.Amazon.com; *www.BN.com*;
www.deepershopping.com, and
wherever books are sold.

To order directly from the publisher,
visit: *www.healthylifepress.com*.
Unless otherwise noted on website, shipping
is free for all products purchased through HLP.

www.healthylifepress.com

For information on our products, or how to publish with us, e-mail: *info@healthylifepress.c*

A Simply Homemade Clean
by Lisa Barthuly, homesteader

"Somewhere along the path, it seems we've lost our gumption, the desire to make things ourselves," says the author. "Gone are the days of 'do it yourself.' Really . . . why bother? There are a slew of retailers just waiting for us with anything and everything we could need; packaged up all pretty, with no thought or effort required. It is the manifestation of 'progress' . . . right?" I don't buy that!" Instead, Lisa describes how to make safe and effective cleansers for home, laundry, and body right in your own home. This saves money and avoids exposure to harmful chemicals often found in commercially produced cleansers.

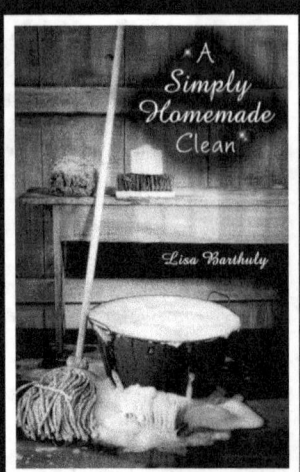

Paperback: $16.99   eBook: $6.99
Both: $22.99 (direct from publisher)

The Secret of Singing Springs
by Monte Swan

The Secret of Singing Springs is a story inside a story that is inside still another story. The book opens with the discovery of an old axe, leading geologist Morgan Russell and his three children on a treasure hunt and transporting them back into local outlaw history starring Jesse James. But the hunt is only the beginning of what becomes an ever deepening mystery, eventually leading to the discovery of something lost that holds the promise of something waiting to be found in the Front.

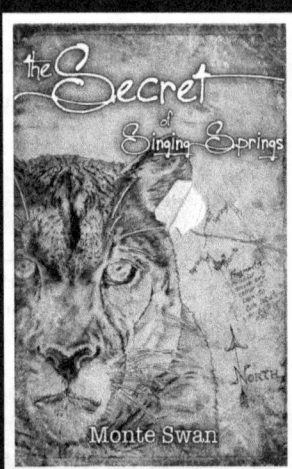

Paperback: $12.99   eBook: $9.99
Both: $19.99 (direct from publisher)

Printed books and eBooks available at
www.Amazon.com; *www.BN.com*;
www.deepershopping.com, and
wherever books are sold.

To order directly from the publisher,
visit: *www.healthylifepress.com*.
Unless otherwise noted on website, shipping
is free for all products purchased through HLP.

www.healthylifepress.com

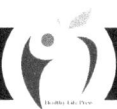

For information on our products, or how to publish with us, e-mail: *info@healthylifepress.com*

God Loves You Circle
by Michelle Johnson

Daily inspiration for your deeper walk with Christ. This collection of short stories of Christian living will make you laugh, make you cry, but most of all make you contemplate—the meaning and value of walking with the Master moment-by-moment, day-by-day.

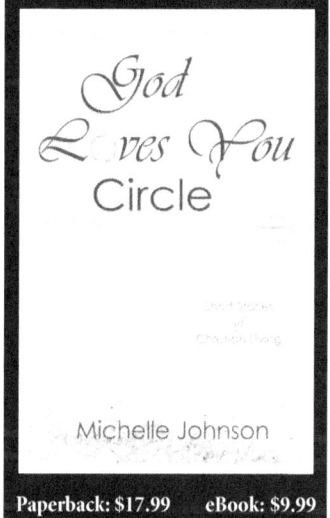

Paperback: $17.99   eBook: $9.99
Both: $22.99 (direct from publisher)

Our God-Given Senses
by Gary A. Burlingame

Learn about your nine senses. Increase your awareness of them in everyday life so that you can better incorporate them into your writing and speaking. Let your senses take you back to Eden and give you hope in the feast that awaits you in eternity. And thank the Lord for how wonderfully made you really are (Psalm 139:13-14). Especially helpful for anyone who often does public speaking or creative writing, including pastors and business people. Creatively suggests ways to incorporate the senses into your communications as a way to draw readers or listeners into your topic and toward a deeper understanding.

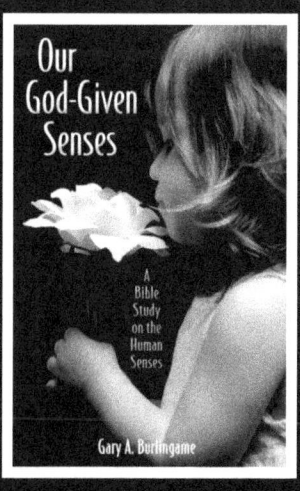

Paperback: $12.99   eBook: $9.99
Both: $19.99 (direct from publisher)

Printed books and eBooks available at
www.Amazon.com; *www.BN.com*;
www.deepershopping.com, and
wherever books are sold.

To order directly from the publisher,
visit: *www.healthylifepress.com*.
Unless otherwise noted on website, shipping
is free for all products purchased through HLP.

www.healthylifepress.com

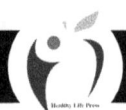

For information on our products, or how to publish with us, e-mail: *info@healthylifepress.com*

Vows
A Romantic Novel
by F.F. Whitestone

When the police cruiser pulled up to the curb outside, Faith Framingham's heart skipped a beat, for she could see that Chuck, who should have been driving, was not in the vehicle. Chuck's partner, Sandy, stepped out slowly. Sandy's pursed lips and ashen face spoke volumes. Faith waited by the front door, her hands clasped tightly, to counter the fact that her mind was already reeling. "Love never fails." A compelling story.

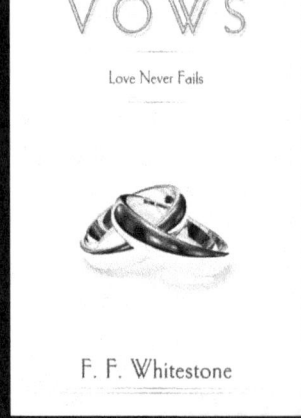

Paperback: $12.99   eBook: $9.99
Both: $19.99 (direct from publisher)

Worth the Cost?
by Jack Tsai, MD

The author was happily on his way to obtaining the American Dream until he decided to take seriously Jesus' command, "Come, follow me." Join him as he explores the cost of medical education and Christian discipleship. Planning to serve God in your future vocation? Take care that your desires do not get side-tracked by the false promises of this world. What you should be doing now so when you are done with your training you will still want to serve God.

"Strategic students know that today's decisions lead to tomorrow's reality. When truth is truth it applies in all contexts. While Dr. Tsai emphasizes his lessons learned as a student of medicine, these insights of wisdom apply to all believers who happen to be students."

– Nick Yphantides, MD
Chief Medical Officer
San Diego County

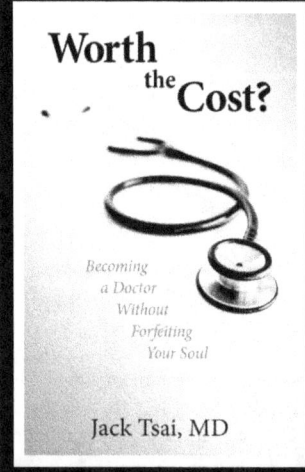

Paperback: $12.99   eBook: $9.99
Both: $19.99 (direct from publisher)

Printed books and eBooks available at
www.Amazon.com; *www.BN.com*;
www.deepershopping.com, and
wherever books are sold.

To order directly from the publisher,
visit: *www.healthylifepress.com*.
Unless otherwise noted on website, shipping
is free for all products purchased through HLP.

www.healthylifepress.com

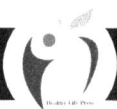

For information on our products, or how to publish with us, e-mail: *info@healthylifepress.com*

He Waited
by LaDonna Cooper

Inspires readers to wait upon the Lord for His best for them; stresses the importance of putting God's purpose above one's own; emphasizes that God's love is unconditional; demonstrates the wisdom of waiting, through a combination of positive insights, encouragement, biblical examples and principles. Decorated with original poetry by the author. For singles and others who are waiting.

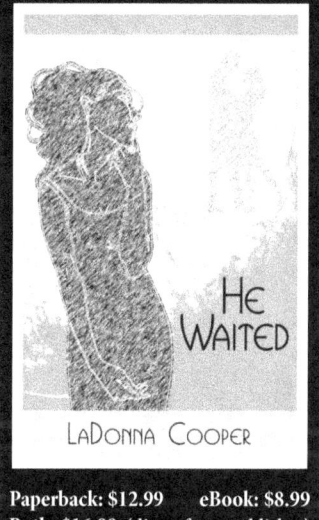

Paperback: $12.99   eBook: $8.99
Both: $16.99 (direct from publisher)

The Big Black Book
What the Christmas Tree Saw
by Rev. Warren C. Biebel, Jr.

An original Christmas story, from the perspective of the Christmas tree. This little book is especially suitable for parents to read to their children at Christmas time or all year-round.

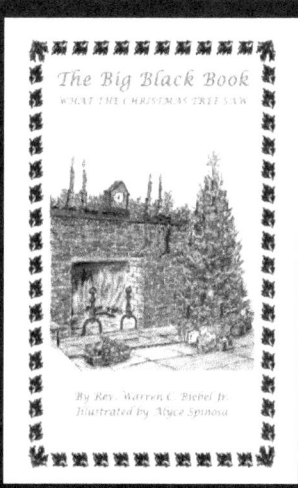

Paperback: $10.99   eBook: $9.99
Both: $15.99 (direct from publisher)

Printed books and eBooks available at
www.Amazon.com; *www.BN.com*;
www.deepershopping.com, and
wherever books are sold.

To order directly from the publisher,
visit: *www.healthylifepress.com*.
Unless otherwise noted on website, shipping
is free for all products purchased through HLP.

www.healthylifepress.com

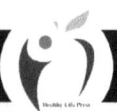

For information on our products, or how to publish with us, e-mail: *info@healthylifepress.c*

ANNOUNCING PEAK PUBLISHING

a new division of Healthy Life Press, featuring resources in printed and/or electronic forms that are for the reader's enjoyment, education, or edification. These resources convey a wholesome, positive message that may not be specifically Christian or even religious.

For information about publishing with us,
e-mail: *info@healthylifepress.com*.

A Midsummer Rose
Once-a-Week Tips to Energize Your Life
by Ashley Coplen

In the style of CS Lewis and JRR Tolkien, this author's first novel features spells, curses, prophecies, dragons, potions, werewolves, vampires, a wicked witch, and a wise wizard. Get ready for intrigue, mystery, danger, and romance as a fair young maiden and a handsome prince overcome impossible odds to fulfill their destiny.

Published by Peak Publishing
(A Division of Healthy Life Press)
eBook only at Amazon.com for Kindle; or
www.healthylifepress.com for ePub or PDF.

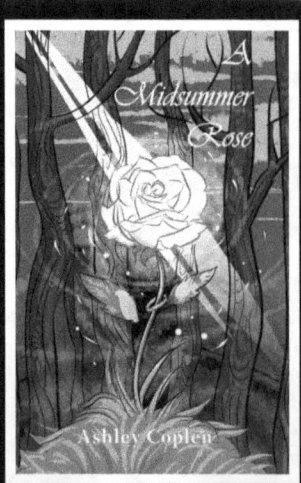

eBook: $9.99
ePub/PDF: $9.99
(direct from publisher)

Printed books and eBooks available at
www.Amazon.com; *www.BN.com*;
www.deepershopping.com, and
wherever books are sold.

To order directly from the publisher,
visit: *www.healthylifepress.com*.
Unless otherwise noted on website, shipping
is free for all products purchased through HLP.

www.healthylifepress.com 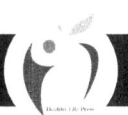 For information on our products, or how to publish with us, e-mail: info@healthylifepress.com

About Healthy Life Press

Healthy Life Press was founded with a primary goal of helping previously unpublished authors to get their works to market, and to reissue worthy, previously published works that were no longer available. Our mission is to help people toward optimal vitality by providing resources promoting physical, emotional, spiritual, and relational health as viewed from a Christian perspective. We see health as a verb, and achieving optimal health as a process—a crucial process for followers of Christ if we are to love the Lord with all our heart, soul, mind, AND strength, and our neighbors as ourselves—for as long as He leaves us here. We are a collaborative and co-operative small Christian publisher.

For information about publishing with us,
e-mail: *info@healthylifepress.com*.

Printed books and eBooks available at
www.Amazon.com; *www.BN.com*;
www.deepershopping.com, and
wherever books are sold.

To order directly from the publisher,
visit: *www.healthylifepress.com*.
Unless otherwise noted on website, shipping
is free for all products purchased through HLP.

www.ingramcontent.com/pod-product-compliance
Lightning Source LLC
Chambersburg PA
CBHW071601080526
44588CB00010B/981